Love Your Disease

LOVE
YOUR
DISEASE

It's Keeping You Healthy

John Harrison, M.D.

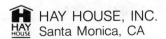
HAY HOUSE, INC.
Santa Monica, CA

Dedication

for
Dr. John H.M. Rudolfer, teacher and fellow explorer.

When there were no words left,
I remember him dancing.

Contents

Acknowledgments

To Kar Fung Santaro-Wu I give thanks for my early acupuncture teaching, but more importantly, for her personal unaffected demonstration that balance and beauty were really possible. She did not teach me Yin and Yang, but then, she lived it. On my return to Australia, Dr. Rudolfer spent four years treating me, deprogramming me from ten years of medical school, teaching me dietetics and refusing to accept standard notions of cause and cure. From him I learned to shift my frame of reference and to risk doing something different. Although we now differ in our respective treatments, we share a fundamental understanding of people's needs, the most basic of which is the need for love.

When I was still searching, I found Graham Andrewartha and Susan McPhee to help me through the transition phase of unwillingness to accept personal responsibility, and through them I was introduced to the new psychotherapies—Transactional Analysis, Gestalt, Radix, Bodywork, Encounter, Hypnotherapy,

Psychological Level Communication, etc.

For the psychological theory which I have applied to the cause and cure of physical illness, I thank Eric Berne, and before him, Freud. My teachers have included Kristyn Huige, Bob and Mary Goulding, George Thomson, Steve and Carol Lankton, Harry and Laura Boyd, Jeffrey Zeig and the aforementioned Graham and Susan.

I have taken the paradox of Yin and Yang and applied it to the psychotherapies, concentrating more on physical illness than on psychological states. From this has emanated a personal perspective on the value of the psychotherapies and, perhaps more significantly, when to quit them.

I am indebted to Humphrey McQueen for his enthusiasm about the original idea and his reading of the manuscript, Geoffrey Farr for his criticism of the theory and his fearless confrontation of my own issues confusing it, and John Emery for his support and assistance with the dialogue.

I would also like to thank the fellow members of my clinical training group who have shown interest in discussing the ideas and, in particular, Peter West for his comments on the manuscript.

Finally, I am grateful to Llyn Smith, who not only provided an intellectual springboard for many of my ideas over the years of the book's formulation, but cared for our son while I was writing it.

Love Your Disease

Introduction

(My disease) went away of its own accord after some years, and I've never had an itch of it since. And I know why. Because I have no further use for it.

My Mask, Norman Lindsay

Disease is both self-created and self-cured. How and why we give ourselves illnesses will be examined in great detail in this work. Having established the ways in which we contribute to the development of our own diseases, we will go on to investigate the ways in which we can minimize our discomfort and, if we so desire, eliminate our disease entirely. The decision is ours. The delightful thing about such a concept is that you, the patient, can once again assume control over both your disease and your destiny. When we become familiar with our investment in developing diseases, we will see that we alone can decide whether to maintain a disease process, allow it to progress, or end it. We will examine the reasons for some people being too scared to become self-responsible, and see how healing ourselves can be great fun—not only fun, but an opportunity to reorganize our whole lives, learn about ourselves and our environment, understand our children and, perhaps more importantly, prevent disease in both ourselves and our offspring. In doing so, we will have practiced true preventive medicine, and understood the most fundamental principles governing health and disease. Illness is the physical and psychological result of unresolved needs, not a malfunction of a machine caused by unknown or external factors. The client is needy, rather than sick, and has exercised an honorable option available to him to take care of himself as best he can. How different an approach to the practice of medicine this is! Rather than merely visiting a medical practitioner with a specific complaint or set of symptoms that we wish removed, we can use the presence of the disease to learn about ourselves and why we've found it necessary, at this particular point in our life, to become ill. We then use our present illness to prevent others. When we are prepared to understand why we have made ourselves ill, we will have taken that first giant leap towards the resolution of our problem. We make use of symptoms, for they are the physical expression of our problem, and to remove them indiscriminately is to dispose of valuable evidence. New physical symptoms will simply replace those hastily removed without reference to the underlying needs that created them. Removing the symptoms does not deal with the needs. We will find the good things that come our way from having a disease and hence understand our reluctance to part with it. The following brief example will serve to introduce this idea.

Peter Walker came complaining of migraine headaches. He reported that they were worse at home, in the evenings and at weekends. For years he had been unsuccessfully treated with medication, and more recently with acupuncture and chiropractic. He was a gentle sort of man with a job in the Forestry Department. His hobbies centered about plants and wildlife and he spent as much time as he could engrossed in journals and books on the subject. His wife was by nature more gregarious, and was generally annoyed at his wish to be alone. She tended to pursue conversations, only desisting when he was clearly in pain. For this purpose his migraines proved ideal.

When Peter Walker learned that he was paying for his wish to be alone by having migraine headaches, he resolved to tell his wife what he wanted instead. He no longer needed the headaches, therefore he removed them. In turn, she decided to stop feeling guilty about going out and enjoying herself and, having satisfied her need for interaction, reported a favorable change in her relationship at home.

When we have established our investment in creating and maintaining our disease, we can decide to achieve the advantages (and these may include attention, solitude, love, respite from work, and others) in less painful and less damaging ways. That is, we can learn to get what we want without needing a disease to justify getting it.

Were a patient to go to a doctor and be given a drug, or to a surgeon and have an organ removed, he would be temporarily symptom-free, but none the wiser—and on the return of the disease, or the development of complications, as impotent as before. The treatment of disease by powerful suppressive drugs and by surgery guarantees the development of further disease. We will examine the reasons behind the "quick-fix" symptom-removal therapy of today.

Introduction

In order to see the mechanisms behind the prevention, development, maintenance and treatment of disease, we will need to look at developmental psychology. In doing this we will trace those factors influencing our health, from conception through pregnancy, childbirth, childhood (the period of diminished responsibility), the transition period (denied responsibility), adulthood (self-responsibility) and parenthood (shared responsibility).

In accompanying me through these pages you are invited to become aware of the role you are playing in your own health, join in the anticipation and excitement of self-discovery, heal your own body and finally rejoice at a celebration of yourself.

THE NATURE
OF DISEASE

1

Factors Influencing Disease

This book concerns itself with the most important and the most ignored cause of all illness—ourselves. Paradoxically, we make ourselves ill in order to take care of ourselves the best we can. The fact that disease is largely under our control, and a physical response to our internal needs, does not deny that other factors are involved. Of course they are. The following chapter examines some of these other factors and shows how even they are partially under our control. Although they are potentially damaging, it's we who determine, usually subconsciously, whether we will fall prey to them. In discussing them, I don't dismiss them but place them in a position secondary to our own investment in being ill or well. We can either use them to facilitate our disease or protect ourselves against it.

GENETICS

There are many textbooks available on the subject of genetics and a discussion of all but the most elementary is beyond the scope of this book. Some diseases are passed from generation to generation with mathematical certainty. Such a familial disorder is classic hemophilia, where half the sons of carrier mothers will have the disease. Females are usually unaffected, as are the sons of affected males. The daughters of affected males will all be carriers. Even in this classically inherited disorder, the degree of bleeding has been lessened during dental extraction using hypnosis, indicating that genetic factors are not the only factors involved. Many diseases *appear* to be inherited. Some of these are governed by the laws of genetics with greater or lesser mathematical certainty and predictability (as with hemophilia), and in these cases parents can be informed as to their chance of producing affected offspring. As a preventive measure, they may decide not to have children because the chance of the child developing the familial disease is too high.

Many more diseases that are seen to afflict families are not governed by the laws of genetics. Some of the commonly known chronic diseases, for example, arthritis, hypertension, asthma and breast cancer, are in this category. If the disease is common among the adults, the children run a greater risk of developing it. For example, if a mother had asthma as a child, and hay fever as an adult, her child may develop the same maladies. The likelihood of this occurring will be heightened if the father also suffers from these diseases. Why?

The answer is to be found within the living and eating habits of the family, and in the role disease plays in the family psychodynamics, that is, how diseases facilitate social interaction among members of that family. Take the following example.

Mrs. Cason brought her eldest son, Peter, aged twelve, to see me because he was suffering from chronic asthma. She was enthusiastic in her praise of the fortitude he displayed in dealing with what she described as "a very debilitating disease for a young man to have to bear." During the interview, he sat quietly, spoke briefly of his desire to go into the air force like his father, and at the time showed the usual physical signs of asthma. Mrs. Cason had been a nursing sister before marrying, and felt most wanted when she was helping others. Her own uncle had suffered badly from asthma and the whole family would take turns to nurse him in the days before bronchodilators and antibiotics. Peter's brothers Simon, eleven, and Andrew, five, had no sign of the illness. While the father was away, which was often the case, Peter would sit at his place at the table, take over his chores like cutting the grass, and often keep his mother company while his two brothers played. During these times Peter would often develop asthma. This suited his mother, who liked caring for her eldest son while he was ill. She was frightened of the tenderness of her feelings towards the boy, whom the local butcher had referred to only last week as her "second husband." She had laughed at the time, and been proud to note how he was certainly turning into a fine young man.

Asthma in the Cason family was an acceptable disease. For generations it had enabled some members of the family to care for the others. It enabled Mrs. Cason to express her love for her son who was missing his father. She was afraid of her sexual attraction towards the boy and felt safer when he was ill. He took care of his mother by providing her with a sick patient to care for, the thing she did best. Everybody had an investment in the disease continuing. Father reinforced it by praising his son for looking after his mother while he was away. In this case the family psychodynamics maintained the disease process.

We will see later how the personalities of children are influenced by their parents and how, in most cases, parents give to their children the messages that they were given themselves. Hence, certain personalities are encouraged within families, and illnesses, we will come to learn, are an integral part of personalities.

In addition to psychological factors, diet and lifestyle tend to be passed from generation to generation. The diet of the father is generally the diet of the son, although in recent times this has changed in the Western world.

Predispositions to diseases are often not passed on in a physical sense (that is, through transmission of faulty genes), but rather through the messages parents give their offspring and the living habits and diet they pass down. The medical profession spends much more time and effort in investigating the physical aspects of disease than the psychological factors. This is as true of the transmission of diseases as it is of the orthodox profession's mechanical view of cause and cure. It seems laboratory data are much more acceptable to contemporary Western scientific thinking than psychological profiles. Personality and behavior are passed most assiduously from parents to their offspring. Given long enough, the components of personality, if reinforced sufficiently, may find physical expression within the structure of genes and may eventually be inherited—like blue eyes. All of nature is a cycle. Psychological states can alter the physical body, and physical characteristics will be reflected within the psyche.

An individual who is angry has a raised adrenalin level. If such a person fails to resolve his anger he will alter his external appearance. The face will show discontentment and may be ruddy in complexion. He'll walk and talk like an angry person. There are also internal consequences of the unresolved anger, such as chronic elevation of the blood pressure (hypertension) and shut-down of the blood vessels in the hands and feet (peripheral vascular disease). All systems and organs of the body are affected by one's psychological state. The testes (in men) and ovaries (in women), carrying the genetic information, are two such organs. After a period they may subtly adjust to the interior milieu of their hosts, thereby passing components of the parents' psychological state to the children. Anger then becomes inherited.

The concept of biological feedback or cybernetics introduced here in simple form will be referred to continuously as we examine how we can use those diseases, which cause us anguish, to help us. This epitomizes my basic medical philosophy, referred to as Paradox, Eternal Change, or Yin and Yang.

CONCEPTION

Many factors influence the ability to conceive. Many others influence the ability to conceive healthy offspring.

A. Rosenbloom, in *The Natural Birth Control Book*, Aquarian Research Foundation, Philadelphia, 1977, has documented that in some peoples, females do not conceive, despite multiple partners over a ten-year period, until they have married and it becomes socially acceptable for them to conceive. In this interval they use no contraception. Such a situation highlights the fact that conception and contraception are under mental control. This control has been largely lost to women in Western society. Many women believe, however, that they will conceive when the time is right for them, and they do. These women are more in harmony with nature's cycles, often ovulating and menstruating in accordance with the moon. When such a woman does not wish to become pregnant, she influences her body chemistry to such a degree that conception becomes impossible. If conception does occur, then spontaneous abortion will follow.

Such a case needs to be distinguished from those in which the woman professes not to want a child and becomes pregnant anyway. I have found in interviewing such women that they were fulfilling parental messages to become pregnant at that particular time. These influences are very powerful and may override even the most unsuitable current social circumstances. Hence large families may continue to get larger in circumstances of poverty, or when the mental state of either parent seems least able to afford it.

Similarly, we all know of cases where a woman is unable to conceive despite years of trying, and both she and her spouse have been given a clean bill of health. In these cases there's nothing physically amiss with either partner, but the woman has some deep-seated fear of pregnancy. She may feel, for example, that to conceive a child would detract from her femininity, that she would cease to be attractive to her husband and that he might leave her. If she has been told by her mother that when a woman has a child she becomes unattractive or less sexy, she will most likely have picked for a husband a man who shares those views. The threat of him leaving will then be quite real, reinforcing her decision in childhood that to have babies threatens a marriage. Under these circumstances it's unlikely the woman will conceive despite all the latest medical technology. Therapy then centers around resolving the fear of the social consequences of childbearing.

I have also found many examples in my medical practice of women failing to conceive until they have spent several months on a dietary regime preparing themselves to carry a child. They are afraid to produce offspring whose health, they argue, may be adversely affected by their smoking cigarettes or drinking tea, coffee and alcohol. After some months on a diet designed to eliminate toxins from their body and supply the necessary vitamins and minerals, they feel confident of conceiving a healthy baby and become pregnant. In those cases, despite clearly wanting a baby, they are satisfying a more deep-seated need to become very healthy themselves before conceiving.

Any system in the body needs to be exercised appropriately if it is to function properly. This is as true for the digestive system, where underuse in prisoner-of-war camps caused later problems, to overuse of the musculo-skeletal system resulting in muscle strain or torn ligaments. In a similar way the reproductive system can be improperly exercised. In the male, sexual excess in the form of too frequent ejaculation may deplete the stores of viable sperm, or deplete the physical reserves of the man so that abnormal sperm become more prevalent. Conversely, an ambitious man may so concern himself with the worries of business that high anxiety levels, combined with a lack of sexual stimulation, may cause low sperm count. In either case, infertility may result.

In the case of females, psychological stress often results in an inhibition of ovulation, or a complete suspension of menstruation. In many others the regularity of the menstrual cycle is upset by emotional factors. Nearly all women will have experienced the effect of anxiety on the regularity and the nature of the menses. Often periods are more painful (dysmenorrhoea) or the blood loss is greater (menorrhagia) at times of emotional stress. Those women who have unresolved tensions concerning femininity, sexuality or conception will often experience an increased level of anxiety immediately prior to menstruating. This is the much-written-about, and little-understood, "premenstrual tension." There are certainly physical changes in the tissues, a consequence of the woman's own attitude to her menstruation. I do not intend here to discuss this detailed topic save to include it in those factors affecting the ability of the woman to conceive, or to conceive a healthy child. Failure to conceive is dealt with at length in Section II—Finding the Cause.

A woman needs to be in a state physically and mentally conducive to conception. It is necessary, for example, that her sexual functioning be active. To enhance this she might surround herself with sexually attractive males and females who are unafraid of their own sexuality and who'll accept hers. She might have sexual intercourse with or flirt with people who arouse sexual desire in her. She will have orgasms from masturbation and mutual masturbation, and just prior to the ejaculation of her male partner she should become readily aroused and have sufficient vaginal lubrication not to require artificial lubricants. The joy of orgasm insures the correct muscular contractions of the pelvic muscles and the correct electrolyte balance throughout the organs of conception. These matters require attention many months before conception is planned. They all contribute to the organs of conception functioning at their peak at the time pregnancy is desired. They represent correct functioning of a system that needs to be exercised like any other. (Who would deny the sense in an athlete training to peak physical condition before an important event?)

In addition to the female achieving a well-functioning genital tract, she needs to alleviate many of the usual burdens of living for several months prior to conception. Financial matters and business problems should be minimized. She needs to feel confident that, having eliminated other commitments, she'll be able to cope with motherhood. Ambivalence at the time of conception results in the mind and body not acting as a unified whole, thus increasing the chances of birth deformities and parental distress.

Before attempting pregnancy, the woman particularly, but also the man (both to help his partner and for healthy sperm production) need to be on a specifically formulated diet. This diet convinces the woman that she's physically fit to become a mother (as we've seen in the cases cited earlier) and balances the body chemistry. Particular attention must be paid to the elimination of drugs, for example, nicotine from cigarettes, caffeine from tea and coffee, tetrahydrocannibol from marijuana, and artificial colorings and flavorings. In the male, alcohol, caffeine and nicotine have been shown to decrease sperm quality. The patient is also instructed in which foods will supply the necessary proteins, carbohydrates and fats. Attention is paid to mineral input, especially calcium, and to the fat and water-soluble vitamins. The diet must be interesting and appealing to the taste. It must be properly presented. Much of this common-sense diet will continue into the gestation period.

PRE-NATAL ENVIRONMENT

Once conception has occurred, the environment within which the fetus will spend the next nine months of its life becomes a major factor shaping its health. Cradled within the womb, it's extremely sensitive to both the physical and emotional state of the mother.

In the first three months of the gestation, referred to as the "organogenetic period," the cells of the embryo are dividing and multiplying so rapidly that small changes in the blood chemistry of the mother may cause significant changes in the direction of fetal growth. Within this period of rapid growth, the conventional medical profession advises caution in the administration of any drugs. They still, however, prescribe antinauseants in large doses to thousands of women, despite the disaster of thalidomide. When, by their own crude assessment, a drug appears to cause no obvious fetal abnormalities, they feel able to recommend its use, although we have neither the biochemical expertise nor the long-term statistical evidence to support or denounce the use of many drugs currently used in pregnancy. My belief is that when the medical profession's tests become more sophisticated (remember this branch of medicine is in its infancy), we'll be able to demonstrate dangers from all drugs taken in pregnancy. I believe that no drugs should be administered in pregnancy, particularly within the first three months. Included within this category are antinauseants, caffeine (tea and coffee), nicotine (tobacco), tetrahydrocannibol (marijuana), narcotics, antihistamines for hay fever, or any others. I believe that even drugs which cannot be shown to cross the placental barrier between mother and child still have an effect on the developing fetus. They do this by altering the maternal hormones which do cross the placenta, as well as by interfering with placental function itself. In addition, many of the complaints of early pregnancy, such as morning sickness, may be effectively treated by natural methods without recourse to drugs. Apart from the imprudent administration of drugs by the medical professsion, many other factors affect the biochemistry of the mother and, indirectly, the child.

The diet of the mother is an important factor. Proper diet can improve the likelihood of conception and it's no less important during the period of gestation, particularly during the early months. Because this is the period of rapid growth or change, the fetus is vulnerable. Common sense is the element lacking in most dietary regimes. It doesn't make sense to me to ignore the vitamins and minerals available in nature and take a pill instead. The general dietary regime in pregnancy needs to provide a balance of vitamins, minerals, proteins, carbohydrates and fats, while augmenting those substances on which the fetus makes a special demand, particularly calcium and iron.

Eating extra dairy products is not the best way to increase a pregnant woman's calcium intake. Drinking twice as much milk to account for the baby's needs often upsets the digestion of the mother, causing bowel and liver disturbances. In turn, the extra calcium in the food is not digested. Some authorities would argue that people who eat few or no dairy products have similar calcium levels to those who consume a great deal. A more radical minority (C. Shears, *Nutritional Science and Health Education*, Downfield Press, Stroud, UK, 1976) suggests that dairy products, high in calcium themselves, may actually remove calcium from the body. An abundance of calcium is available in many cooked vegetables, for example, cabbage, dandelion, turnip greens, spinach, broccoli, kale and parsnips. Nuts, legumes, fresh fertilized hen's eggs, raw oats, indeed any whole grains, also contribute significant amounts of available calcium. Rhubarb, dates, apricots, raisins, oranges, prunes, peaches and figs generally contain lesser but worthwhile amounts. Goat's milk products (milk, yogurt and cheese), with some cow's milk, may be used sparingly.

Vitamins must be taken in the form of a great variety of raw vegetables and, to a lesser extent, raw fruit. The greater the variety, the greater the chance of including all the required vitamins and minerals. Green raw vegetables cannot be successfully replaced by vitamin pills, fruit or any other substance, as their chlorophyll is clearly required in a fresh state. The crisp and colorful vegetables give pleasure to the mother, and foster her desire to create and nurture the fetus.

Those substances which are living, for example, freshly picked vegetables and fruits, and those foods capable of growing, for example, brown rice and the legumes (soy beans, lentils, lima beans, red kidney beans), are more likely to nourish the developing fetus. If a substance is capable of supporting itself (plant a grain of brown rice and it grows), then it's capable of providing a unique combination of vitamins and minerals necessary to sustain us. If a food rots when planted (like white rice) then it cannot support itself, and is unlikely to offer humans the range of essential ingredients we require.

The mother needs to be mentally stimulated by her food. It must be appetizing and well presented. By consuming a very large variety of foodstuffs, not only are the various food categories better balanced, but the maternal digestive mechanisms are fully exercised. This means the fetus develops within a fully functioning human being, whose fluctuations in adrenalin, insulin and other hormones guarantee its own capacity to be fully functional.

In addition to the mother's diet and the drugs she

consumes, other chemicals affect the fetus. The carbon monoxide from motor vehicles, industrial gases, deoderants, perfumes, soaps, toothpastes, the water supply, dyes in clothes, sunscreen applications, washing powders and so on may all be absorbed into or onto the mother and affect the developing baby. Electrical stimulation from electric blankets, radio, television, microwaves and overhead power lines may also be significant. There are many other hazards in the environment with which the fetus must contend. All of these may be disease-promoting on the one hand, and health-promoting on the other, depending on the amount or dose. For example, small amounts of brewer's yeast, one-eighth of a teaspoonful twice a week, supply the B group vitamins, but a tablespoonful taken every day may cause excessive fermentation in the intestine and actually remove vitamin B from the body. A controlled exposure to a substance may easily be dealt with by the fetus and help it to overcome a larger dose next time. An overdose of the substance may cause irreparable damage and subsequent disease developing in childhood or much later in life. However, appropriate exposure to environmental stressors, both physical and psychological, guarantees the quality of life, for we flourish in proximity to those things which are potentially dangerous.

Those factors affecting the developing fetus that emanate from the psychological state of the mother fall within an area that has not received a great deal of attention in the past. Recent development of sophisticated monitoring of, for example, fetal heart rates, hormone levels and state of sexual arousal shows that the fetus is indeed reacting to the emotional climate. An increase in fetal heart rate accompanies maternal anxiety. If this is prolonged and severe enough, the newborn child will already have a stress problem, which may cause it to seek stress situations in the future because of its physiological familiarity with high adrenalin levels. People become hooked on adrenalin just as they become hooked on tea. Such a situation, if perpetuated or expanded by parental messages in childhood, may have serious consequences on the long-term health of the individual.

Recent photographs taken *in utero* have shown males to have erections. This may be a response to maternal sexuality, mediated via placental hormones, maternal hormones or direct nervous system stimulation. The answer will no doubt be provided one day by the physiologists. In the meantime, we may reflect on how a mother who feels very sexual about pregnancy, childbirth and breastfeeding will be affecting her son's or daughter's sexuality. This is neither good nor bad. Whether it will be a positive or an adverse influence will depend on the "dose" and the method of delivery. If the mother is truly delighted to be pregnant, watches in awe and excitement as her abdomen and breasts grow, and expresses a full range of emotions while carrying the fetus, the baby has a great chance of being born without the abnormalities and already "well adjusted."

The father's role in the *in utero* psychological environment is also significant. By providing assistance, love, care and physical comfort to his partner, he can help her to feel safe and well. Another woman can also fulfill this role. In addition, the partner of the pregnant woman can, by speaking softly and reassuringly, accustom the fetus to his or her voice. During childbirth and early infancy this may be of great value in comforting the infant.

Similarly, anger, fear, sadness and joy can be openly expressed by both parents before the fetus is born. These are all legitimate, healthy emotions, and if expressed rather than suppressed will acclimatize the growing fetus to a series of muscular stresses, hormonal states and sensory stimuli, which will facilitate the child's own developing ability to deal healthily, physically and mentally, with a full range of emotions. Having experienced its mother in a full rage, and having witnessed this state passing into a state of calm, the fetus is learning the value of emotional expression while still in the womb. As the fetus develops and experiences its mother in all of the four major emotional states, the fetal systems become capable of responding to emotional demands. This will be valuable during delivery and provide a measure of emotional flexibility with which to deal with the joys and traumas of infancy.

Similarly, sexual activity during pregnancy is necessary. Intercourse, until discomfort or womb instability dictates otherwise, may be continued. Great care should be taken not to contract venereal disease. Masturbation, preferably with a partner, will accustom the infant to the particular movements and sounds associated with orgasm. A later chapter will discuss how a full range of emotional expression is a necessary prerequisite of a healthy body.

If, as is often the case, the mother is in a state of anxiety during pregnancy, the baby will be affected. Misinformation will often cause a young mother to be apprehensive about childbirth. An unsatisfactory relationship may result in a constant state of anger about the pregnancy. In these cases the fear and anger aren't healthy immediate emotional states, but old "leftover" feelings that aren't healthy for the fetus. This is because they are not fully expressed but rather dealt with internally by the mother, resulting in changes in her muscles and organs. A chronic state of tension leads to all manner of bodily complaints. In the case of a pregnant woman, blood flow or metabolic transfer across the placenta may be altered, jeopardizing the well-being of the fetus. There may be no obvious physical abnormalities in a child born to a mother who has been under great stress in pregnancy but as time goes on, various behavioral difficulties, which seem to have no explanation, may arise. These can often be traced back to the emotional state of the mother during pregnancy.

If her partner's voice initiates a chronic fear or anger response in the mother, so too will it affect the fetus. Similarly, a loving partner's voice will be a source of comfort to the developing fetus. The mother's pleasure in relating to other people will condition the emerging infant to do likewise and significantly affect the child's ability to socialize. A mother who feels and shows joy towards her developing child by massaging her abdomen lovingly and by speaking in soothing and welcoming tones will be encouraging her child to be born. Combined with a positive attitude towards the pregnancy by her partner, this will result in a child who has no doubts about its right to exist. Cradled for protection inside the womb, a child grows secure in the knowledge that it's loved and wanted. This knowledge is the greatest gift parents can give. Without it, the tendency to develop diseases is virtually guaranteed.

CHILDBIRTH

Imagine what it must be like to come from the security, warmth, darkness and comfort of the womb into the noise, bright lights, confusion and harshness of a delivery room. Most of us did that, and if we could recall it, would say it was the single most traumatic event of our lives. If the experience was a particularly severe one, as in the case of a forceps delivery or a difficult breech birth, or if the conditions of the delivery environment were very unsympathetic, the fear associated with our own birth may be concealed in our subconscious forever. We'll see later how the power of conditioning depends upon both the impact and the frequency of the experience. In the case of childbirth, the experience is not repeated, at least not physically. The degree of trauma involved may, however, be enough to affect our personalities. Therapies such as rebirthing and primal therapy provide ways in which to "relive" the birth trauma, and by re-experiencing the fear, neutralize it.

Any emotion is legitimate. Any emotion that is suppressed or not allowed expression until it is naturally exhausted will remain embedded within the psyche of the individual and will cause both physical and psychological changes. Childbirth in natural circumstances would leave no lasting impression on the child. The fear of birth and the sadness and anger at leaving warm, known surroundings will disappear within the arms and at the breast of a loving mother. The reassurance of a voice fondly recalled from intra-uterine times will ease the fears of the newborn, and reassure it of continued support. If a child's fears are not allayed by its parents, a decision will be taken by the child. Where circumstances prevent immediate contact between the child and its mother following birth, it may make a very early childhood decision that its needs will never be met, initiating a lifetime of anxiety.

The popularity of soft birth is being justified by the appearance of less traumatized babies. These babies appear to have less adjustment problems, that is, they are more emotionally expressive, more content, surer of their right to exist than other children. The major factors are a positive expectation on the part of the mother, that is, a balance of fear and excitement, which varies according to the number of previous children the woman has had. Many books have been written on the subject of birth without violence, some of which are listed in the bibliography.

Warm support from the woman's partner, soft lights, warmth, placing the child on the mother's breast, cutting the cord after pulsations have ceased, and not violating the child with suction hoses all contribute to the impression of this new world as a nice place to be. A newborn's fears about being able to survive in the new and frightening environment will be allayed by such treatment, and a major decision for health will have been made, the decision to exist.

2

The Childhood
Basis of Disease

Most commentators, psychologists and the public alike agree that the period of early childhood up to the age of six years is the most important in the shaping of an individual's personality and destiny. Within this period the first three years are probably the most significant. The messages a child receives in the first six years of life will largely determine whether the person is a dancer or a dietitian, is married or single, has four children or no children, has diabetes, cancer or dandruff, is homosexual or heterosexual, plays football or smokes a pipe. The parents are more important in the early years while the influence of siblings, peers, relatives, friends and the media increases later on. Decisions the child takes in these early years will also directly or indirectly influence every other aspect of that individual's character and lifestyle, determining even old age or an early death. Such is the vulnerable and impressionable nature of early childhood. As this book is about our state of health, we will be concentrating upon those messages promoting either well-being or illness. These same messages affect our social lives and the ease with which we achieve peace and happiness.

Those people who are generally happy to be themselves and who satisfactorily resolve childhood conflicts (even though inadvertently) will be healthy. Those who are unable to accept themselves and live with guilt, fear, anger, anxieties, doubts and sorrows will eventually develop physical diseases. An infant's mind is virgin territory. Every single incident is unmodified by experience, and therefore profound. As we become older and more experienced, individual incidents have less impact on us because they are modified by those before them.

Factors affecting personality, health, disease and the curing of illness have their greatest impact during periods of change. During gestation, childbirth and early childhood we are in such a state of change and these times become crucial periods of development. Why are children so impressionable during those early years? It's because they are unsure that they can survive, and therefore they adapt to the wishes of the "big people" in their lives who are capable of keeping them alive.

Consider the following: You're reading a book entitled *Love Your Disease*. It's keeping you healthy. You've found the opening remarks to be interesting, and you're looking forward to uncovering more reasons why you may be continuing to make yourself ill. You decide to settle down comfortably for a couple of hours and keep reading, since the book is very readable, and you know that in two hours you'll have covered much of it and have understood its relevance for you. The benefits appeal to you.

Now consider this scenario: You begin to feel a little cold but you can't put on more clothing or turn on the heater. Perhaps you're a little warm but you can't take off your clothing or turn on the air-conditioning. You're slightly uncomfortable but haven't the strength or the skills to lift a cushion into place. You're hungry but haven't the coordination or the mobility to fetch something to eat. You're thirsty but unable to get yourself a drink. You're scared because you can't keep yourself alive and you want somebody to hold you. Let yourself *feel* what that might be like.

What do you do? How do you get someone to help you? What must you do in return, in order that the help might continue? What needs of yours are you prepared to sacrifice to be cared for by those about you who can help? What is the cost to you? What do you decide to do in the future?

Such needs, inabilities, fears, pressures and decisions face the baby every day. Because the child is inexperienced, he will not know what is safe, and because he's unable to care for himself, he will make decisions upon what he perceives to be dangerous. In order to feel safe he's receptive to parental demands and hence, if father is better disposed towards him when he doesn't cry, the child may make a decision not to cry. Of course, father may not physically harm the child if he does cry but at this stage the child doesn't have that information. The incorporation of this early childhood message, "Don't cry," has sown the seed for later psychological imbalance and ensuing illness, for later we will see how a failure to cry may result in sinusitis.

In the animal kingdom, many of the young can protect themselves, at least to some degree, in the first few months of life. A calf may, by running away, evade a minor predator in the first few hours of life. Other birds and animals may be protected by armor or camouflage. By comparison, human babies have no physical protective mechanisms. Indeed, if a baby were left on its own below the age of two years, it probably couldn't survive. Physically defenseless humans protect themselves, or try to feel safe, by using their intellect. This is as true for the infant taking great notice of the "big people" about him and assessing what they require of him, as it is of the mature adult in his or her conquest of stronger animals.

The baby, contrary to common belief, is very receptive to parental pressures. It's finely tuned to the emotional state of its parents and other members of its family. It monitors their anger, sadness, fear and joy and, by the age of six months, can be seen checking out many things it does with a quick glance at its caretaker. While it is incapable of caring for itself, it needs to be aware of the responses of those who guarantee its survival. The infant's thinking capacity is, however, immature, and so some threats to the baby will be perceived, rather than real. This awareness is much more developed than its physical coordination, which makes the baby appear to be either not reacting to what's going on around it, or to be crying indiscriminately. Vulnerability forces the baby to react to parental pressure. This vulnerability has a number of components.

Being so small, the infant lacks power. Parents are usually at least one-hundred times stronger than infants and, in conjunction with their much larger physical bulk, leave no doubt in the baby's mind as to who would win a physical showdown. Siblings, even though they may only be a few years older than the infant, are nevertheless much more physically competent and able to support their point of view with brute strength if necessary. Fear of physical pain motivates an unconvinced infant to comply with a parental or older sibling demand or attitude. At such an immature stage of development, the infant is unable to handle stress adequately and, in order to avoid stress coming its way from the parents, may choose to behave in certain ways. If mother becomes upset when a small girl placed in the bath begins to masturbate, the girl will most likely respond by stopping the practice and "taking care of mother." By taking care of her own caretaker, the child is effectively taking care of herself. The child is in no position to confront much parental behavior and hence acquiesces with the parental viewpoint. Mother may, in order to relieve her own sexual anxiety about masturbation, offer the girl some toy to play with. If this situation is repeated often enough, the child may take the decision that masturbating is wrong or harmful and will later on experience anxiety in similar situations. In this she has followed her mother. Because masturbation produces such pleasant bodily sensations, the child may believe that mother doesn't want her to do anything that makes her feel good. This may not be what mother wishes to convey at all but because of the child's immature thinking capacity, that may be her response. This decision could have disastrous effects in the future, resulting in an individual unable to physically "feel" pleasant sensations.

The resultant lack of stimulation to the surface of the body contributes to an imbalance in the internal organs, a concept recognized in acupuncture and Eastern medicine. A belief central to acupuncture is that the internal organs are represented on the surface of the body by meridians or channels of energy. If these body surface points are not stimulated regularly, then an imbalance is set up in the internal organs, which later results in organic disease, for example, gallstones or stomach ulcer. Similarly, contemporary psychology has shown that lack of adequate physical stroking of the infant can result in serious psychological disturbances both in children and in adults. Hence, for the healthy development of the child, both for the growth of the internal organs and to let the child know it is loved and wanted, much cuddling and stroking of the whole body is advisable. It's also enjoyable for the parents.

An infant hasn't the experience with which to balance or quantify a message. It hasn't the information with which to reject certain data. If a child is indirectly told by a parent that she is dumb, for example, by overhearing the father saying to the next-door neighbor, "She's not as smart as her brother," she may decide, "I am dumb." As a child she doesn't understand that her father may have an investment in women being dumb, whereas if she were older and overheard a similar statement, she would have the information to reject it: "That's just the old man's chauvinism speaking." Hence, lack of information in childhood may result in children accepting information about themselves that they would reject in a neutral situation. They are not, however, in a neutral situation. Their view of the world is adopted from their parents, and, more importantly, their view of themselves is similarly influenced. In these circumstances the child has few options, the best of which is to go along with the beliefs of the parents. However, despite the lack of available options, it's still the child who is making the decision to comply or rebel. At a later time, an adult may choose to alter some of those early childhood decisions in order to cure himself of disease.

We have considered some of the reasons why children are susceptible to the influence of parents and other big people in their lives. These messages, the positive and the negative, are acted upon by the child and incorporated into his personality. The combination of these decisions and their related behavior is the individual's personality. Because messages need to be repeated and delivered with authority to be incorporated into one's personality, the parents clearly influence the young child most, although the media and other people become increasingly important as the child is able to understand more.

We will consider next the nature of these messages and the mechanism whereby they are finally transmuted into diseases. To do this, we will use some of the theory of Transactional Analysis and Gestalt psychotherapy, as these disciplines describe the early childhood decisions clearly. One form of message coming from the parents is "injunctions." These are described as "a prohibition, or an inhibition of the free behavior of the child." They reflect some of the deepest fears, angers, sorrows, and desires of the parent. They may be given directly or indirectly, verbally or nonverbally. The injunction "Don't be a child" is one commonly given to the first-born child in a family. Inexperienced parents are often frightened of harming very young children and are only too happy to see them grow quickly and become more self-sufficient. Such a child may decide he is unworthy of the love and caring he sees his younger siblings receive from parents who now feel much safer about babies. As an adult he may continue to deny himself love, believing caring and affection to be for others who are more deserving. On the other hand, the last-born in a large family may be given a "Don't grow up" injunction, often when mother has enjoyed child-rearing and wants to prolong the experience. Such a person may marry late, remain closely attached to his parents and choose a partner who treats him like a child. These individuals frequently suffer acute illnesses, which bring their partner scurrying to their aid, a situation that suits both of them and which they learned in childhood. The major injunctions and their opposites, permissions, are:

Injunctions	*Permissions*
Don't exist	Exist
Don't feel	Feel
(emotions,	(emotions,
sensations)	sensations)
Don't think	Think
Don't be close	Be close
Don't be you	Be you
(that is, a boy or a girl)	
Don't be a child	Be a child when a child
Don't grow up	Grow up when ready
Don't make it	Make it as you want
Don't do	Do what you want

The first of these, "Don't exist," is called the primary injunction. The rest are really modifications of "Daddy doesn't like you climbing over him, dear," Mother may inform young Peter, which is indirectly saying it's only OK for you to exist if you don't climb on Daddy. All of the injunctions are a modification of the right to exist, which the child interprets as meaning his continued existence is only guaranteed if he satisfies certain parental requirements. In the case of a powerful and often repeated message to not exist, the child may take the decision that death is the best option. He may then exercise that option by having a fatal accident, or by dying of leukemia. (But not all children who die young have "don't exist" injunctions.)

Where either parent doesn't want the child for any reason and communicates this to the child, that child will grow up with a "don't exist" injunction. The strength of the injunction will depend on the frequency and power with which it is given. A casual comment to the effect that Dad was not altogether ready to become a father when Susy was born, will probably be of little import, especially if it's obvious that he now loves her. At the other end of the scale may be a father who continually berates a child for being born and subsequently ruining his business and social life: "If it weren't for you kids, I'd be wealthy by now." In this case the child may assume responsibility for his father's unhappiness and decide his father would be better off if he, the child, were dead. He may act on this belief in a number of ways, consciously or subconsciously, mentally and physically.

When a parent says angrily to a child, "I wish you were never born," the child has the option of believing, Mom wishes I were dead, or maybe, Mom's upset, she doesn't really mean it. In the first instance, the child has furthered his script (that is, his personal life plan decided upon in response to parents' messages), and in this case has consolidated his belief that he wasn't meant to be alive. In the second example, the child has already decided that it's OK for him to exist, and rationalizes his mother's hasty remark.

If someone believes "I shouldn't exist," then certain events are made more likely. He neglects to protect himself against dangerous or life-threatening situations. These people may engage in dangerous sports (motorcycle racing, daredevil stunts). They may join the armed forces and apply for active duty, or become mercenaries. They may become involved in dangerous occupations like illegal drug-trafficking or, in some parts of the world, become policemen. Not all people in the above categories are trying to fulfill their parents' messages to not exist, but dangerous occupations do attract people who are ambivalent about living. So does cancer.

Most people who decide that their parents didn't want them and who subsequently don't take all available measures to stay alive, do not become mercenaries. Instead they may drive their cars dangerously, fall asleep at the wheel or drive under the influence of drugs or alcohol. In these ways they put their lives at risk, getting a real thrill from flirting with death, often with tacit parental approval. When these people eventually seriously hurt themselves or kill themselves, we all cry, "What bad luck, to have a fatal accident at such a young age!" But often that was no accident. Why did the young woman, apparently enjoying life and with a successful career, fail to notice the bald tire on her car? Or if she noticed it, why didn't she take the time and effort to have it changed? Why did the handsome young lawyer fail to notice the oncoming bus as he stepped from the curb? These people weren't trying hard enough to stay alive. In other words, they had manifested their early childhood decision to "not exist" and exploited available hazards to effect that decision.

There are other ways to act on the parental injunction "Don't exist." Illness is one of these. An option for everyone is to end their life by giving themselves a fatal illness. Bear in mind that these decisions to die are mostly taken subconsciously. A person rarely says, "Life for me is intolerable, I'll give myself cancer and die." However, if the mind is giving the body too few messages of the "keep healthy, stay alive, stay sane" kind, then the potential for physical illness exists. How does this happen?

Various glands in the body (adrenals, thyroid, ovaries, testes) are under the control of hormones produced by a gland in the brain called the pituitary. These glands in turn produce substances that profoundly affect the functioning of the body. The pituitary gland is affected by our psychological state. When we're afraid, the adrenal gland produces adrenalin, which dilates the pupils, increases the heart rate and causes us to sweat. This prepares the body for "fight or flight." What is happening to us emotionally will be simultaneously affecting us physically. Imagine the physical effects upon the body during a lifetime of these chemical substances (hormones) circulating in response to us thinking and feeling about ourselves in certain ways. All of us are able to look at another person's face and see anger, joy, sadness or fear, which in some cases has been so longstanding as to cause permanent changes in the facial features. This may happen at quite a young age, so that the person may look like a "bitter young man." Emotions that are left over from childhood and not resolved (racket feelings) are as capable of altering the internal organs as they are the facial muscles. Eventually, the physiological effect will cause anatomical changes, that is, the psychological state is transformed into physical disease. So what's new? Most people believe that anxiety causes stomach ulcers and emotional upsets result in intestinal upsets. But this thesis goes beyond stress, for here

I am explaining both the origins and the advantages of stress. Acting upon the messages given to us in childhood, we see ourselves as someone with an unqualified right to exist, a qualified right to exist or no right to exist. Over a period of time, our mental attitude affects our body chemistry (physiology) and keeps us healthy or, in the case of those with a powerful "don't exist" injunction, eventually kills us. That is, we kill ourselves. Hence people may develop a life-threatening disease such as cancer or prolong an otherwise innocuous disease like hepatitis, until they die from it. As in the case of the road "accident," the fatal illness has merely followed their instructions to their bodily functions, and killed them. This will usually be subconscious. For a person with this belief, life becomes intolerable. By dying, he fulfills his most fundamental belief: that he has no right to exist. Not many people have such a powerful "don't exist" injunction but many have modifications of it, injunctions intended to keep them alive but which modify their behavior. We will be looking at these shortly.

As the child becomes an adult, he'll often decide to change that early childhood decision. He may do this unwittingly, alone, with friends, a spouse, by joining a psychotherapy treatment program, or in many other ways. An important point about the injunctions is that they are not usually given in a direct way, and indirect messages are often more completely absorbed by the child. That's why people who have given themselves life-threatening illnesses, when invited to recall such messages as "We don't want you" are often genuinely unable to do so. They were never given directly. Let's look at some ways in which parents give their children indirect messages and see what the child makes of them.

Take a situation where the younger of two boys is being bullied by his older brother. The younger child is in real need of physical protection and the only way available to him is to get someone to look after him. Because of greater availability, he may choose his mother. She may invite the child to become ill or weak in order to protect him from the older boy, the bully. The illness justifies her repeated berating of the older boy who is, of course, jealous of his newly arrived brother: "I told you to stop bothering your younger brother. You know he's not as strong as you." Now this message, given not to the boy himself, but to others, or even only implied by the mother's protective actions, offers the younger child the option of being protected by being ill. As he grows older, he may be less anxious when he has some ailment than when he's perfectly well, for when he's in good health he may feel unprotected and vulnerable. The role of illness in this case is to invite the protection of other people.

Those messages that define or label a person are called "attributions." They are very powerful because children are presented with a statement about themselves in which they have no say, a *fait accompli*. "Oh yes, he's not as sturdy as his brother," Mother reports to an inquiring neighbor, thereby recommending frailty to the child. It's thought by many people that attributions (statements made about the child indirectly or often simply implied by the parents' actions) are the most powerful of all parental messages. A common example with which most of us will be familiar: "You're just like your father/mother."

The whole family may contribute to the disease process in one or more members of that family. Our young boy who became ill to get his mother's protection was pressured into doing so by his older brother, invited to use that option by his mother and covertly supported by his father who chose not to intervene. The interaction between members of a family will often initiate and maintain both health and disease. In some families, disease is simply unacceptable. In others, family members have permission to suffer "nervous breakdowns," but no physical diseases. The ongoing interaction between members of a family is referred to as "family psychodynamics."

There are other categories of messages given by parents to their children. Some of these are called "drivers." These are messages that restrict the child's free behavior. They often represent messages given by parents wanting to make the behavior of their children socially acceptable, and therefore help the children be successful in life. As such, they're often effective, resulting in a successful businessman, for example. At the same time they may lead to much anguish as the person struggles to maintain a lifestyle based upon them. Illness is often a consequence of the drivers, as demonstrated in the following example:

A forty-three-year-old man was to be transferred to a new appointment in a city some 800 kilometers away. His wife wasn't keen on leaving her friends and voiced strong opposition to the move. Not wishing to upset his employer, the man agreed to go but was suddenly struck down with gout, a condition which he'd suffered only once before, some ten years previously. As the new position involved increased traveling, the employer sent a younger man instead. By giving himself gout, which was the physiological result of his wish to be immobilized, the man justified staying where he was, rather than follow his driver of "Please me" and continually seek promotion as his father had wished.

This example shows how effectively illness can result from, and then be used to break, early childhood messages, rather than the individual taking responsibility for breaking them. The matter of personal responsibility in illness will be taken up later.

The opposites to drivers are "allowers":

Drivers	*Allowers*
Be perfect	Be yourself
Hurry up	Take your time
Try hard	Do it
Please me	Consider and respect yourself
Be strong	Be open and get your needs met

The child is coerced by fear into following the driver directives. The child perceives parental disapproval for not following the drivers as a threat to his own existence. What the parent is saying or implying to the child is that he's OK only so long as he's perfect, hurries up, tries hard, pleases the parent or is strong. If the child does not fulfill these parental wishes, then he risks loss of parental strokes, love and support. To a young child, this is life-threatening. We have spoken before of the balance of power between infants and adults and I think it bears repeating, for only by understanding the pressures upon the child to conform is it possible to see why people are prepared to give themselves diseases. When they do this, they are following decisions they have taken in childhood at a time when it was prudent to do so. It is essential for anyone who is ill to acknowledge that they have decided, at some stage, to contribute to their disease. Only then are they powerful enough to take the decision to remove it.

As we get older, many of the decisions we took in order to be looked after best as children are no longer relevant. We can now look after ourselves and need neither parents' approval or support to do what we want, nor an illness to justify breaking an earlier parental directive.

Many of the drivers are messages which, if taken up by the child, result in successful people. Those who possess the personality traits of perfection, strength and urgency often make excellent professionals, business people, public servants and trades people. If they fear losing parental love for failing, they'll often be unhappy and eventually give themselves a serious disease. This is a consequence of both the physical strains of fulfilling the directives and the advantage of contracting a disease in order to justify breaking them. Such is the paradoxical nature of the cause and cure of disease.

It's possible for parents to raise successful children who aren't driven by fear. Allowers, as the name implies, are a category of parental attitudes facilitating self-determination in children. They are listed opposite their driver counterparts. The allowers encourage children to do things for their own benefit, rather than for the benefit of their parents. This removes the urgency of achievement and fear of failure and, in so doing, promotes mental and physical health.

The development of disease from driver behavior is interesting. Before we examine that, however, we need to understand how the personality of the individual develops from these various messages—the injunctions, attributions, drivers, permissions and allowers. An injunction or attribution is incorporated into the personality only when the child decides that he'll accept it, that is, the child decides to not exist, to not be close, to be a member of the opposite sex. This decision is taken under duress. Nevertheless, it is still the child who is making the decision. When the decision has been taken, the injunction or attribution is incorporated into the script. The script is a personal life plan decided upon by an individual at an early age in reaction to his or her interpretation of both external and internal events. Hence:

INJUNCTION / ATTRIBUTION + DECISION ⟶ SCRIPT
(Given by Parents, etc.)   (Taken by Child)

The child may decide to incorporate the drivers into her belief system. This series of decisions becomes the subscript. Hence:

DRIVER   +   DECISION ⟶ SUBSCRIPT
(Given by Parents)   (Taken by Child)

The script and subscript usually mutually support each other, and are the basis for thoughts and feelings about self that promote the development of disease.

The mechanism of disease development from driver behavior is varied. This is because no two individuals have the same script or subscript even though there are familiar patterns. When genetic factors, environmental factors, age and other variables are taken into account, it can be seen that a strong "be perfect" driver may result in a heart attack in one patient and a stomach ulcer in another. Often this is because certain diseases have been given a degree of acceptability within families or communities. Heart attacks, for example, are common in the menfolk of some families and unpopular in others, who may consistently suffer gout. Diseases, like table manners, are modeled by grown-ups. If, as a child, a boy hears about Grandpa who "worked himself to death" in the family business, and Uncle James who had a "mental breakdown" and was forced to retire, the boy may decide that if work becomes too onerous, disease is an acceptable way out. If the family scripting or modeling is coupled with a "be perfect" driver, the boy may end up giving himself a disease. "We had such high hopes for Trevor, he had distinctions in both years of his economics degree, but now that he's been unfortunate enough to become schizophrenic, who'll run the company?"

At a later date, should the disease become sufficiently irritating, the discomfort may motivate the person to face the fear of, and then break, the original decision. When he has decided to be well for himself and not simply to remove the discomfort, he'll no longer need the illness, and in this state of self-responsibility can attain good health. Using one's current illness is a good place to start and constitutes the transitory advantage of disease.

There is another component to driver behavior. People incorporate drivers into their subscripts because of a fear of parental reproach if they don't. The only way to alleviate the fear is to continue to drive yourself. This, as we have seen, alters the body physiology and eventually causes physical changes. Hence disease may result from unresolved fear, anger or sadness. We will examine this more fully in Section II, Chapter 6. Drivers are often associated with societal values. C. Steiner in *Scripts People Live*, Bantam Books, New York, 1974, says: "The subscript is an acquiescence to the cultural and social demands that are transmitted through the parent."

Disease must be looked at in a cultural as well as a personal and familial setting. In contemporary Western society, disease is commonly an end result of a script. People who remain in script are essentially non-self-responsible, since they are continuing to observe parental directives. They don't believe they can, as adults, please themselves, and similarly don't believe they can protect themselves from physical diseases which they, like society generally, attribute to bad luck. Having suffered the disease, they may then use it to stop pushing themselves. If they assume responsibility for giving themselves the original condition and decide to stop making themselves ill, they will have changed their script and started on the road to health.

Consider the following sporting "accident": I ruptured my Achilles tendon playing squash. If it hadn't been for this injury, I'd have been a champion. Now I won't be able to realize my full potential. Of course, if my full potential wasn't as good as my parents had hoped, then I would have been a failure in my eyes. I may or may not have been a failure in my parents' eyes, depending on whether my childhood perception that I needed to be perfect in order to get loved by them was correct. This injury serves to relieve the anxiety of not being perfect. Now I can enjoy my squash at a much lower level of achievement, more consistent with my ability. "Be perfect," you will recall, is one of the drivers. Such people strive for success until eventually they do themselves physical and psychological harm. And of course, if a person always strives for more, they're never content with what they have, irrespective of their level of achievement. A person with a "be perfect" driver is trying to achieve or retain his parents' love by being a perfect person. There are, of course, gradations of "be perfect": I could have prevented this injury by deciding to play at a lower level of stress before I gave myself an injury.

Illness is a physical and psychological consequence of the script and subscript and involves any permutation of drivers, injunctions and attributions. It is prevented by the allowers and the permissions. These are the *personal* causes of illness. In addition, there are numerous *external* causes of illness, for example, genetics, womb environment (physical and psychological), childbirth, environmental pollutants, diet, physical activity. Some of these are under our control, others are not. We may use them to facilitate becoming ill.

The physiological processes responsible for converting psychological states into physical disease are being increasingly studied. Research conducted at the University of Sydney by a psychobiologist, Dr. Dale Atrens, in 1980, produced some interesting information. Obese people who attempt major weight reduction by dieting are often frustrated after an approximate five percent weight loss. This is because the brain resets the circulating blood levels of thyroxin and adrenalin at a lower level, thus reducing the basal metabolic rate and preventing further weight loss. This is an automatic response of the body to maintain the pre-existing weight and is not dissimilar to hibernation.

I believe these individuals subconsciously decide to remain obese, even though they may be dieting. Subconsciously they instruct their pituitary hormones to maintain the old weight until such time as they feel safe enough to be slimmer. Then they lose weight with minimal or no dietary change.

Physiognomy, the diagnosis of psychological states by facial appearance, is practiced effectively by all of us. One of the least true things my mother told me was that people can't help what they look like, in reference to someone I found unattractive. People's faces reflect their personalities exactly.

The physical consequences of scripting can reasonably be expected in the internal organs in much the same way as they can be seen in the face and body. Script issues may find expression in disease if left unchanged. I believe a man who as a boy has decided to be non-sexual (different from a "don't be a boy" injunction), will often have a smaller penis than his father. Similarly, small breasts or amenorrhoea may be indicative of a sexual injunction in a woman. These things can be changed.

The injunctions "don't feel emotions/sensations" may lead to an individual who fails to spontaneously express fear, anger, sadness or joy, and this in time affects body physiology. The injunction may only cover some of the emotions. Some parents are very happy to have their children express joy but not anger, for example. It's interesting that in acupuncture, suppressed anger is claimed to cause liver disfunction and suppressed fear is said to result in kidney malfunction. I believe both to be true.

Visualize for a moment a dog experiencing the joy of his master's return. The furious wagging of the tail and the movement of the whole spine stimulates both the central and peripheral nervous system and balances the internal organs. This is a basic tenet of Chinese medicine: the well-being of the internal organs depends in part on what happens to the external body. Touching, stroking and sexual stimulation all energize and regulate the function of the liver, spleen, kidneys, lungs, intestines, heart, gallbladder, urinary bladder, pancreas and the thermal and chemical regulators of the body. Hence, a person who does not get themselves touched is inviting physical disease.

Physiological imbalances may arise as a consequence of not directly expressing emotions. Where rage, for example, is suppressed, there may be a chronic elevation of adrenalin leading to hypertension, a flushed face and eventual cardio-vascular pathology. Sinusitis is an example of a condition that is often caused by people (usually men) refusing to cry. The resultant swollen and chronically inflamed mucous membranes would have returned to normal had the person shed tears at the moment of sadness. I speculate that if emotions were spontaneously and totally expressed then body physiology would be temporarily exercised and rapidly return to a state of healthy equilibrium. In a similar way to exercising the biceps, a good cry or yell will keep the body functional. What are some of the "advantages" of illness? Many people will not change script decisions because the little kid in them is afraid to do so. When the pain or suffering of the disease is greater than the fear of the original adaptation, they may change. That is to say, the pain of illness, itself part of their script, may prompt them to overcome the fear of changing the original script decision. They may make their illness responsible for change. This may have been specifically incorporated into their script or subscript; for example, a heart attack in a businessman with a "be perfect" driver may have been considered by his parents a valid reason for slowing down at work. Having made himself aware of this, the businessman may decide again to make himself responsible for how hard he works and discard illness as a way of giving himself permission to slow down.

The advantages of illness are illustrated in the following: "People get ill to get what they want (caring, etcetera)" and "People do not get what they want (caring, etcetera) so they become ill."

We will be looking at the prevention of disease, using healthy early childhood messages, in some detail in Chapter 20—Healthy Parenting.

3

When You Go
to the Doctor

A client I was seeing for the first time told me that she'd known of the work I was doing some nine months before coming to consult me about her medical problems. I found this information surprising, considering the progressive and debilitating nature of her illness. "Why," I asked her, "did you wait for such a long time when you knew your friend who recommended me had made a dramatic recovery from a similar condition?" "Because I was scared you would insist that I change the way I was," was her reply, "and I wasn't sure I wanted to do that." In the meantime, this woman's condition had deteriorated substantially, yet her fear of change had obviously been such that she preferred to live in pain. Only when her symptoms became physically intolerable did she come for treatment.

This interesting attitude led me to ask all my new clients how long they had waited before coming to see me. The average time was about four months. Since they had all heard from whoever had recommended me that I worked on removing the disease by eliciting the personality factors behind it, I assume their reluctance to come indicated that they were afraid to look closely at themselves.

Now, this I can understand. If a person has made a decision in childhood that turns out to be counterproductive later on, they will have done so because of fear: fear of losing something more important to them than the inconvenience of modifying their original behavior. For example, it is better not to cry when you fall over and hurt your knee and thereby obtain Dad's love and approval for being brave, than to cry (which is what you'd like to do) and risk censure.

The same fear that caused the original adaptation leading to or contributing to the illness will be evoked as soon as somebody (in this case me, the therapist) wants to begin "poking about in the past," as one client expressed it. Such a way of expressing it is significant because it shows the anger that very often overlies the fear of looking back. In general terms, people's physiology becomes disturbed and leads to illness not when they express fear, anger, sadness or joy but when they repress those emotions. In the case of the woman who didn't want her past "poked into," it was fear of the fear that maintained her illness and therapy centered around making her feel safe enough to risk confronting her fears. When she was no longer afraid to do things which directly benefited her, she was on the way to a cure. Because of fear, which is really the infant's fear of not being loved and therefore not surviving, people will push unwanted feelings and thoughts to the backs of their minds and expend an enormous amount of time and effort in doing so. This is what so often leads to the lack of energy that many patients complain of. It's not the result of insufficient sleep, excessive work, poor diet or lack of exercise but a consequence of needing to keep the mind and body hyperactive so as to avoid unwanted thoughts and feelings. The alternative is to express our feelings freely, to laugh heartily when we're happy, cry when sad, yell when angry and have wide eyes, a fast pulse and start to sweat when afraid. To do this has major physiological benefits and is energy-restoring as opposed to energy-depleting.

Anybody prepared to make fearless decisions in their best interests will avoid all major illness and most minor ones as well. Some people, through lack of information, will predispose themselves to problems, for example, eating foods low in fiber, like white bread, and thus suffering from constipation before they discover that fiber is necessary for good bowel function. However, most people who suffer from constipation are fully aware of the need for dietary fiber but ignore the information. By so doing, they use their illness for other, secondary gains and only allow solutions to their problem to enter their awareness when they no longer need the illness. This is the way they have learned to look after themselves best, by using illness, and this is not a bad thing. A small percentage of people will become aware of the role of illness in their lives, be prepared to risk doing some things differently and dispense with the need for illness altogether. In general, relief of physical constipation will rapidly follow relief of mental constipation. Flexible minds make flexible bodies, capable of adjusting to environmental change.

There are two features of becoming or remaining well that between them provide a balanced approach to whole-person health. The first of these is the willingness to take responsibility for our own safety and the second is the willingness to risk.

We take care of ourselves by ignoring, selectively suppressing or simply not noticing those things in ourselves and others that challenge our view of ourselves. For example, if I consider myself an excellent doctor and most of my clients seem to get well, then I may ignore the fact that people who have difficulty expressing their sadness don't do well under my treatment. The reason for my failing to notice this is that I'm not prepared to look at my own sadness, because I do not feel safe doing so. If I'm unprepared to confront my own sadness, it's unlikely I will be effective in helping others confront theirs. Now, in this I'm looking after myself, which incidentally is a good primary rule for therapists as well as clients. Those clients who do not get what they need from me will seek out another therapist. It's a cornerstone of my thinking about why so many patients accept bad and ineffective treatment from doctors that people choose the doctor and the treatment they want, that is, they choose *for themselves* what seems to *me* bad and ineffective treatment.

We keep ourselves safe not only at an unconscious level (as in the previous example) but also by being aware of things that we are simply not prepared to do. Many people could benefit considerably from a change of lifestyle and diet and, although they know this, choose to continue with their current living habits and are prepared to accept responsibility for their decision. Clearly they view the disease they are suffering from as less of a problem than changing some other aspects of their lives. This is a valid decision and I consider that we all do the same thing, at various times and with varying degrees of awareness. How much we choose to care for ourselves physically at any one time is very flexible and will depend upon our current psychological state. When we drop the old fear, our minds will instruct our bodies to function harmoniously and beautifully. Before we drop the fear we aim to have our adaptations reinforced, and it's in this frame of mind that we may go to the doctor.

The humorist who said, "If surgeons performed the operations on themselves that they perform on their patients, there would be far fewer surgeons and far more patients," had more than a cursory appreciation of the dynamics between patient and doctor. However, the truth is that there are the exact number of surgeons operating that the community is prepared to support. When people decide that they no longer require operations, then the number of surgeons able to make a living will fall accordingly. At any given time, the popularity of various medical practices and philosophies rises and falls. The forces that change medical practice come predominantly from the medical profession reacting to a more general movement in society, not from doctors making unilateral decisions. When an individual doctor such as myself decides that the basis of disease lies in childhood and that we manipulate our state of health rather than the reverse, it is because that doctor has been looking at his or her own life. The methods available for this task are a reflection of the collective psychology unique to the early part of the 1980s in Western society. As such they are effective for those people living in that society at that time and less effective elsewhere. The advances in medicine will reflect the willingness of people to look at themselves and their problems from a different perspective. This inevitably involves some risk-taking.

When people buy goods and services, they enter into a contract with the seller; that is, for an agreed amount of money the goods change hands or the services are rendered. In the majority of cases, the contract is not written and may not even be verbalized. It is nevertheless understood by both parties and agreed upon before the transaction takes place. Failure to acquaint oneself with the fine print of the contract, whether it be verbal or written, is often the reason why one party ends up dissatisfied with the transaction and why both parties may end up in court.

We tend to contract in our personal relationships as well, although this is usually done subconsciously. This is not a written contract in the majority of cases or, if it is, as in the case of the marriage contract, the contract only covers the absolute legal essentials. The main part of the marriage contract is unwritten, is quite different in each marriage and often ends up in disarray through failure to clarify it early on in the relationship. As in the case of goods and services, both parties may become confused or disillusioned with the contract and may end up in court. A contract between long-standing friends may be broken when one has an affair with the other's partner, although this has never been discussed as a clause in the contract and neither has mentioned it as a reason for ending their relationship.

In a similar manner, a contract is drawn up between the patient and the doctor. This contract is generally not stated and is never written. The contract states that the doctor, in exchange for money, will remove the unpleasant symptoms that the patient is complaining about. In much contemporary practice, where a patient refuses responsibility for his own illness, the contract states that the doctor will not remove the disease process by recommending anything disruptive to the patient's chosen way of life, will tell the patient what he wants to hear rather than what might help him, and will guarantee the continuation of the disease process albeit in an altered form.

As in the case of the other contracts, this one will last only as long as it suits both parties. If the doctor repeatedly decides that the antibiotic requested by the patient is not necessary, then the patient will most likely change to a doctor who agrees with him and is prepared to prescribe the requested drug.

Every disease we give ourselves has advantages. The advantages lie in helping us to maintain a belief system about ourselves, others and the world which, although damaging to us in some way, effectively masks more deep-seated and fundamental fears. By becoming ill, we spare ourselves the trauma of examining those aspects of ourselves we have chosen to suppress. When disease is regarded like this it becomes clear that if the doctor attempts to instruct the patient in the true nature of the disease, in most cases the patient will become scared and will resist or redefine the information. If the doctor persists, then the patient will seek alternative advice and the doctor will lose the patient and the money. Thus in most medical practice the contract between the doctor and the patient covers only the removal or modification of the symptoms. Provided the doctor is effective in removing the symptoms quickly, which usually means using a powerful drug, and provided the patient on his part does *some* of what the doctor suggests and also pays his account, then the contract remains in force and both parties remain satisfied. This form of treatment guarantees the continuation of the disease because there's been no attempt by either the patient or the doctor to look for the cause.

Let's look at some interaction between patient and doctor that offers evidence of the real nature of the contract between them. I have indicated that the patient is expected to do only some of the things that the doctor prescribes or suggests. In the past few years, a new aspect to the selection and prescription of drugs has been developed which deals with patient compliance, that is, the degree to which the patient takes the doctor's advice including the drugs prescribed. To the naive observer, the degree to which most patients comply with the doctor's advice appears remarkably low. The reality is that virtually no patients comply completely with the doctor's advice. The reasons advanced for this are all rather scientific and ignore the most obvious reason, that is, the patient doesn't want to be rid of the disease.

Very few doctors expect their patients to adhere totally to their advice. Experience shows that even when suffering from a particularly irritating and chronic condition, patient compliance is low. Both parties to the contract know that. The doctor says, "Now, Mrs. Jones, we haven't been taking our tablets, have we?" with a knowing smile. Mrs. Jones responds with a sheepish grin. Both she and the doctor know this means, "No, I haven't been taking all the medication and you can be very sure that I won't be taking this new lot either." The contract for "some of the symptoms to be removed and the illness to continue" having been satisfactorily concluded, both parties leave, agreeing to reconvene the meeting at a later date. At that and subsequent visits, the routine continues until the client decides to get better and therefore breaks the contract or the doctor becomes frightened or disillusioned and sends the patient to a specialist. In these ways much, but not all, of contemporary medical practice is conducted. The five-minute consultation, with no chance of really understanding anything of impor-

tance about the condition, and the broad categor-
izations of diseases with their standardized drug treatments have all been specifically developed to cater for
these sorts of contracts. This is "normal" medical
practice.

Looking for the cause of the disease has recently
become the fashionable pursuit of medical practitioners and paramedical practitioners with an eye to
the marketplace. Hence, the burgeoning field of "holis-
tic" medicine, which could have been the great leap
forward but threatens to become lost in commercial-
ism. In order for the idea of alternative and preventive
medicine to become fashionable and marketable, people must be able to feel as safe with the new medicine
as they felt with the old, with the new requirement
that they must feel they have become more closely acquainted with the cause of their problems. The
majority of patients are still very reluctant to look at
how their personality may be contributing to the disease and at how their reluctance to change some aspects of their behavior is maintaining the problem.
Hence, many increasingly popular therapies must *appear* to be earnestly searching for truths, while the patient's investment in maintaining the disease is
ignored by mutual agreement. This is the reality of
many of the alternative healing arts when practiced
narrowly. I do not believe that diet, homeopathy, acupuncture, chiropractic, herbalism, radionics, naturopathy, osteopathy, chelation therapy, orthomolecular
medicine, vitamin therapy, color therapy or any other
of the healing arts, when practiced in isolation and
without regard for the psychology of the client, are of
more than passing value. The same can be said of
orthodox Western medicine. All of these alternative
healing arts can significantly contribute to the well-

being of clients who are in the process of working through their reasons for giving themselves the disease. While in this transition period, which may last from a few hours to several years, symptomatic relief is required by most patients. This is available using any of the modalities listed above, including drugs, and many more.

For a system of medicine to contribute to the healing process and support the body in curing itself from within, it must not be too disruptive of body physiology in its efforts to provide symptom relief. In this regard, many of the alternative healing arts are ideal, and much of orthodox drug treatment is akin to working on a piece of fine jewelry with a pickax. The curative powers of the body work overtime in an attempt to eliminate the massive doses of antibiotics, antihistamines, analgesics, diuretics and aperients administered by doctors too uninformed and frightened to do otherwise, and taken by patients too intent on instant symptomatic relief to consider probing into why they chose to make themselves ill in the first place. While the body is dealing with these artifically introduced agents, it must continue to heal itself. Consequently, a simple complaint that could have been eliminated by the patient in twenty-four hours is often prolonged by the introduction of a drug. A major reason for the continued success of orthodox medicine is its ability to prolong what could have been a simple minor complaint.

Now that may sound ridiculous but it's the logical consequence of our custom of giving ourselves physically destructive complaints in order to manipulate our environment. We are not ridiculous; we harm ourselves physically in order to protect ourselves psychologically. This book establishes that connection, and offers alternatives.

Orthodox medicine and unenlightened alternative medicine, which together constitute nearly all medical practice in the West, prolong illness. They do this by labeling the patient as ill, rather than needy. Thus the patient becomes someone needing expert medical care, which prolongs the victim status and usually achieves the patient's desired ends, that is, offical sanction to ask for help, caring or other things. Without this official medical sanction, many people will not ask for what they want. They were taught in childhood that capable women and strong men don't do that. Hence, the very real need in society for a popular system of medicine compatible with this characteristic of the society, the unwillingness to ask directly for care when it's needed. Disease that is permanently removed by treatment would no longer serve this function, and that's why orthodox drug treatment has perfected symptom relief and basically ignored the causes of illness.

The contract that those members of the public who don't wish to take responsibility for themselves make with the medical profession goes something like this: "I have consulted you to have my need recognized, my suffering validated, my pain removed and my disease retained. In return, I will support you financially and give you status commensurate with the powers I ask you to exercise."

Each part of the contract is necessary to the whole. In order that the expertise and validating power of the doctor may be legitimately sought, people need a disease. This validation is officially recognized by giving doctors far-reaching powers in all manner of things, many of them having little or nothing to do with medical practice. Doctors, for example, may witness signatures for passports and other legal documents, are variably invited to be members of committees and boards within communities and are offered credit cards and other facilities with no questions asked. All these things are intended to keep doctors on a pedestal as it's an essential part of healing and the validation of suffering that they be seen to be powerful. And of course, this prominence also serves to make the doctor more vulnerable to attack.

If the word "disease" is broken into its two parts, it becomes "dis-ease," which means "uneasy" or "uncomfortable." We tend to go to the doctor when we're uncomfortable. Because psychological discomfort is not afforded the same status as an obvious physical disease that can be measured in the laboratory, it's similarly less effective in having our need and suffering validated.

Why, one may ask, is psychological dis-ease regarded as less valid than physical dis-ease? This is an anthropological question that would take a whole book to answer, but it serves our purpose here to look at it in the light of contemporary orthodox medical practice.

In general, the scientific principle has been very poorly applied to the humanities. The scientific principle requires that one researcher's experiments be reproducible; that is, if a treatment works with one person or group of persons then it ought to work, if it's valid, with any person or group of persons—that is, results are predictable. While this works in the laboratory where conditions are standardized, it's highly doubtful if any of nature is identical. This means that even the most scientific of laws are merely descriptive of what is observable *most* of the time. Human beings seem to me the least standardized of all nature (though no doubt a tree or a cat would disagree with me). Most modern doctors like to think they are very scientific because they've been taught laboratory methods of diagnosis and are familiar with the latest advanced technology. Because of this, they welcome measurable physical disease and are frightened by psychological problems. Hence, if the patient wants his suffering to be socially sanctioned, he needs to come up with a physical ailment. Usually the confirmation of illness is a semi-public testament and can be used much like an invalid Social Security card.

The orthodox view that medical practice is "scientific" means that an equally "scientific" (and equally fallacious) treatment may be used. This is effective in removing the symptoms but of no help in curing the disease. And therein lies its value, the maintenance rather than the cure of illness, for you'll recall that an integral part of the contract is the need to be able to show a physical disease. If that's a prerequisite for being helped, then removal of the disease is not required.

This is neither a bad nor a good thing. It is simply what happens a lot of the time when a patient who doesn't want to take responsibility for himself goes to the doctor. There are plenty of people who can ask for help from others when they need it, can take powerful decisions in their best interests and have no need for illness or the doctor. There are also many other people who give themselves relatively minor illnesses and use the ritual of going to the doctor for permission to get better, often *despite* the chemical or drug they administer on the doctor's advice. There is also a substantial number of cases where the person's investment is in being so ill that all the drugs and technology available to modern medicine are required if he is to stay alive. Fifty years ago these people would have chosen a disease *just* capable of being controlled with the techniques available at the time.

The doctor has been a powerful person in most cultures. The form of the healing has varied tremendously but if there is one feature common to all medicine men of all ages and cultures, including our own, it is mystique. Without mystique I believe the healer could not function effectively. Mystique is a careful blend of admiration and fear. It requires the healer to be powerful and to possess greater knowledge and understanding than the recipient. In the twentieth century, an epoch of incredible scientific advancement, the doctor must be seen to be technologically advanced. As soon as the public becomes familiar with X-rays, the doctor needs to be ordering computerized axial tomography. As soon as the public becomes familiar with penicillin, the doctor needs to be prescribing clindamycin. "Needs to" because, without the progression of medical practice to bigger and better things, the illusion is lost and without the illusion the doctor is impotent.

There's a mutually sustaining fear in all of this. The fear on the patient's side is something I have already spoken of in great depth, the fear of taking full responsibility for who he or she is. The fear of the doctor is the fear of not having the answers and of having his or her system of medicine exposed for the sham it is. This sham includes, of course, the doctor. For these reasons medicine has always been mystified. The doctor hides behind technical names and masks of all descriptions while the patient thankfully puts himself "in your hands, doctor."

Similarly, the doctor is placed on a pedestal by joint agreement. It's worth reiterating that all these arrangements can only survive by joint agreement. As soon as one party breaks the contract, the system is replaced by another. Because our society is capitalistic, the doctor has to be well provided for financially in order, once again, to maintain the illusion of potency. This also provides a very convenient avenue for complaining about the treatment a patient has received, or about how the treatment was ineffective. As a spin-off, an outlet for aggression is provided for those who are unhappy and are looking for someone other than themselves to blame: "Doctors' salaries are absolutely outrageous." Those capable of providing the greatest salvation must be capable of providing the greatest anguish. This is the basic paradox.

It becomes obvious from the preceding discussion that the medical practitioner is a highly significant member of our society. The doctor will be different things to all people and people will seek out the doctor they want. Some will use their doctor as a resource center for researching and understanding mental and physical processes. On a purely mechanical level, the doctor has a deeper understanding of pathology than at any other time in history. If the doctor can be encouraged to impart some of this knowledge, it can be effectively combined with a client's understanding of his or her investment in the disease, and help an early resolution of his illness. Similarly, the doctor's knowledge of symptomatic drug therapy can be temporarily valuable. An alternative practitioner of the healing arts can also be of real value to clients seeking to understand their illness, so that they may assume responsibility for it.

Those medical practitioners who refuse to take the onus of recovery from the client onto themselves are doing their clients a great service. Some people who have decided to get well may in the early stages require the permission of a parent figure they regard as powerful, namely the doctor, to oversee their recovery. Placing themselves under the umbrella of a practitioner reduces the fear they experience when they start to take responsibility for themselves. In effect they are using the authority, status and protection of the doctor to override their own parents' messages. This stage of their development I have termed the "transition stage."

Often, however, the doctor is interested only in labeling the disease without any reference to the underlying reasons for it. This will inevitably be a superficial classification based upon obvious symptoms, readily elicited signs and insensitive laboratory data. (Bear in mind the average consultation with a general practitioner takes well under ten minutes.) The administration of a drug conveniently allocated to that combination of signs and symptoms guarantees continuation of the disease and the patient's contribution to it. In a similar way, psychiatric diseases are categorized and then treated with drugs with little reference to the underlying psychodynamics.

This is "care and control" psychiatry and unfortunately constitutes a large proportion of psychiatric practice. Psychotherapy that orientates clients towards an understanding of why they have made themselves ill and what they can do to heal themselves is real psychiatry.

Modern general practitioners are little acquainted with the causes of illness and indeed it would be financially disastrous for them to regard disease as "self-created and self-cured." In addition, their mechanistic and technically orientated training leaves them threatened by the mention of psychological causes of physical illness. In this climate of mutual support for each other's fears, doctor and patient may contract to ignore the patient's contribution to the illness, remove the symptoms and watch helplessly as acute goes to chronic and the disease worsens.

An increasing number of clients are choosing to use the doctor as a resource center, the healing arts as a means of understanding their illness and contract with themselves to remove their illness when it no longer suits them to have it, that is, when they no longer need it. In assuming responsibility for their disease, they assume the power to remove it.

4

Disease—
Misfortune or Advantage?

A notion in our society that is widely held and aggressively defended is that people, through no fault of their own, will from time to time become unwell, may have accidents and may require surgery. Getting ill or staying well is regarded as a matter of chance, misfortune or luck. So deeply rooted in our belief system is the concept of disease as both inevitable and out of our control that in treating disease we usually look only at the very last point of expression of the disease—the symptoms.

Beneath the symptoms, those irritating and unacceptable aches and pains, is a vast network of interrelated causes and factors contributing to the disease. In all but the most enlightened medical practice, these are ignored. Instead, we concentrate on the tip of the iceberg, forgetting the major features of the illness that are unaffected by the treatment and continue to cause further trouble.

We are all familiar with the idea of treating the cause of the disease rather than treating the symptoms. Despite our familiarity with causes and symptoms, the medical profession is still reluctant to investigate beyond the most superficial basis of disease, and the public in turn is equally disinclined to patronize practitioners who aim for a cure rather than an improvement of the disease. And yet to most people the idea of being reluctant to part with disease is senseless. Because of this, the value of disease in our society needs to be scrutinized.

Why do the majority of people become angry when confronted with the part they play in the development of their own illness? Why does the medical profession continue to regard the patient as a victim of disease? Presumably, the idea that we cause our own illnesses must disturb some very fundamental belief we hold about ourselves and our bodies and a challenge to that belief causes great fear. We pass this fear on to our children and they in turn believe that they don't cause their own illnesses.

What are the advantages to us, as a society, in continuing to believe that we "catch diseases" or develop them because of factors beyond our control?

Firstly, disease that afflicts us "out of the blue" exonerates us from taking responsibility for who we are and for what we're doing to our bodies. To put it another way, by maintaining that we are the victims of disease, we reinforce our belief that we are not in control of our own lives and destinies. If we did accept responsibility for every single event in our lives, including our state of health, how would we feel? I think many people would feel very scared.

It's therefore an attractive proposition to most people that if they become ill, it's not their "fault." I put the word "fault" in quotation marks because, along with the word "blame," it contributes only to the discussion by virtue of us excluding it. Both words carry feelings of guilt and shame. Let me state quite categorically that there's no place in the thesis that we cause our own illnesses for the idea that people with illness should feel ashamed or guilty. Quite the opposite. We give ourselves illnesses in order to "take care of ourselves" psychologically, which is in no way reprehensible. As human beings, our quest for less pain, less anxiety and greater happiness is only admirable. If we give ourselves illnesses, that must be a legitimate way of taking account of greater needs. This book examines how and why we give ourselves illnesses.

I return to why we like to think we are the "victims" of disease, that we can neither cause nor cure disease and why we would be afraid to believe otherwise. The answers to many of these questions are to be found within the experiences of childhood. After all, it's here that our first interpretations are made and our first decisions taken. The child lacks power and therefore makes prudent or expedient decisions given a limited range of options. As we get older, these options expand and our early childhood decisions become inappropriate or obsolete. As adults, we can take care of ourselves and no longer need to coerce our parents into caring for us. It's this need to be taken care of by people more powerful than ourselves that leads us into taking some decisions that are damaging to us in the long term.

Take a simple case such as obesity. A young child has certain food requirements that, given adequate exercise, would result in a standard weight range. In some cultures, parents and relatives believe that children should have a large surplus of body fat to be healthy. If the children are of average weight, they are fed excessive quantities of fat-producing foods in order to put on weight and become overweight. The anxiety of the family is removed by having the child overweight. The child, who is very much affected by tension in the parents and family, will do what she can to lessen stress in both herself and her parents. Thus she takes the decision to be a fat child and will often continue as an obese adult unless she decides something different as she gets older. If she's grossly obese, she may increase her risk of heart disease and gallbladder disease, for example. Thus her early childhood decision to be fat, which was effective in reducing anxiety in everybody, is now resulting in potential physical disease as an adult.

Now this case has several interesting components. If the fat girl had decided she was solely responsible for her weight and had chosen to ignore her parents' directives to be fat, she would have risked censure, maybe physical punishment, and perhaps imagined losing other necessities in her life that she was incapable of providing for herself such as love, touching, clothes. Tension in the family may also have increased. As a child, she would be unlikely to handle such tensions with ease. All of the above factors created a situation in which the child decided that to be fat was her best option.

Children are not responsible for themselves. Parents are clearly responsible for keeping their children alive in the first few years of life. In this period, the child comes to rely upon a person more powerful than himself who is capable of solving problems and meeting his needs. After that, the culture of the society will dictate at what rate responsibility is handed to children as they turn into adults. In many societies, there are specific rituals and ceremonies for just this purpose.

Many of our beliefs about ourselves are created in the first few years of life. The belief that we are not solely responsible for ourselves is one of them and, as a child, that is exactly the case. But the decisions of childhood may be carried through into adult life even though they may be harmful to the adult in some ways. The belief that we aren't totally responsible for ourselves and that others will take care of us may be expressed by getting ill. Our investment lies in reinforcing our belief that some things are beyond our control, and illness is accepted by society as being beyond the control of the individual. As a child, things *were* beyond our control.

In addition, if we get ill, we'll be cared for and comforted as in childhood. Childhood was a time of diminished responsibility with the comfort of knowing that there was somebody more powerful to step in and solve the problem. By maintaining our belief that "we couldn't help it," we try to revert to a belief system that existed as a child.

And no wonder we feel afraid when faced with the prospect of being totally responsible for ourselves. As a young child, such a prospect would have terrified us because it would have meant certain death. I point out that if the child had no reason to fear his needs were not going to be met, he would not fear for his own survival. However, if the mother doubted her ability or desire to adequately care for her child, then this doubt would be passed to the infant. A very young or inexperienced mother may feel inadequate when the baby first arrives. This is to be expected. If these feelings continue over the years, and particularly if they are coupled with ambivalence or plain hostility towards the child, then the child may begin seriously doubting whether he *can* survive. He would most probably decide he couldn't keep himself alive, she couldn't keep him alive, and look for ways to get her or others to take better care of him. Getting ill is one way children do this. The depth of this fear can be seen in the fact that people give themselves life-threatening diseases rather than face the fact that they are responsible for themselves.

Many philosophers have written about humankind being ultimately alone. Disease is commonly used by those people who won't believe they are their own final arbiter. In this sense, disease is like a fatalistic religion and anyone who has worked in a general medical practice or a hospital will attest to the comfort many patients feel as a consequence of being ill and therefore getting themselves cared for. For these people, disease becomes a way of life, an essential component of everyday existence.

There's always the opposite end of the spectrum too—those people who take great joy in the power they have over their own lives can fulfill their dreams. These people will be successful in what they want for themselves and will have little need for diseases. They may from time to time suffer acute complaints because of environmental hazards that combine with old childhood messages they have chosen to retain, but they will not put themselves at risk for major trauma or serious illnesses. These people have overcome any fears they had in childhood of not being able to take care of themselves. They will live as long as they want to, usually choosing to die peacefully when the infirmities of old age become intolerable to them or when they've simply achieved for themselves what they wanted. Let us recall the example of the obese young girl who makes herself overweight in order to facilitate the smooth running of the family. There is a further element to this story, beyond that of an obese adult following childhood messages that are obsolete. The family believed a fat child was a healthy child. That sort of belief doesn't arise overnight and has probably been held for generations in that family, that village, that society, maybe that country. And more likely than not, it was a view with much truth at its beginning, which meant that fat babies were more likely to survive than thin ones. Any number of circumstances may have validated that view. If the seasons were variable and the crops could not be relied upon, then through a bitter winter, indeed the fatter the child the greater the buffer against famine.

Now the point is this: the family living in the twentieth century in an affluent society was following old instructions, which were simply no longer necessary. There was no lack of food, nor in the foreseeable future would there be. Therefore, the need to keep babies overweight was archaic and inappropriate. Can we make use of this example when looking at why our society still chooses to give itself diseases?

The parents' messages to the children and the example they set by showing their children how to live their lives will be maintained by community attitudes generally. For example, most parents bringing up children in the 1950s in Western society would have been more antagonistic towards premarital sex, nudity, marijuana and inflation than parents with young children in the 1980s. In addition to the negative messages given by parents to their children on these matters, there would have been few marijuana-smoking nudist parents living out of wedlock who could model these attributes to children, thereby condoning them. The society was of course far less accepting of these traits. In the 1980s the scene has changed considerably, and society is more tolerant of such behavior. The reasons for change will be varied and include the media, economics, politics and maybe the "Age of Aquarius." The end result is that children now grow up with quite different messages from the ones they received thirty years ago because societies and the people in them change.

Is the need for illness fading out, like the need to keep babies overweight, or are factors at play that are strengthening the need for illness? It's surely worth asking why both families and society generally contribute to the child's belief that illness is an acceptable, indeed a much-condoned, way to escape the fear of self-responsibility. Put simply, some people kill themselves by disease rather than face their own power to live or die. Dying surrounded by caretakers is preferable to the uncertainty of existence.

Let us look now at the creation of wellness, using the framework already established in our discussion of how and why people give themselves illness. If the child were given no reason to doubt his survival, he would believe the world to be a safe environment in which his place was guaranteed. Such a child, surrounded by loving caretakers, would believe in his own power to create favorable circumstances for himself, since from birth his experience had been that his very presence induced happiness and pleasure in those around him. He would have no reason to fear that unless he fulfilled certain parental expectations his right to exist might be revoked. Instead, he would become confident that things he did in his own interests would, if not directly help him, then at least not harm him.

Now this is the basis for believing that we're in control of our own lives. We would have no reason to be tentative when doing things in our best interests if

our memory of doing just that in childhood was positive. As adults, we would take decisions in our best interests fearlessly. As a matter of course we would keep
our bodies healthy and free of major trauma or illness.
We would not believe disease was beyond our control
if we had no childhood memories of needing to be ill
or helpless in order to be cared for. Parents who allow
their children to feel powerful by supporting the decisions their children take in their own interests will
foster the belief that the children are powerful and
capable of both preventing and curing illness.

5

Self-Responsibility, Health and Disease

Let's examine what happens when a young child wants something. The newborn cries when she wants to be fed, when she's wet and wants to be changed, when she's cold and wants to be made warm, when she wants to be held, comforted, or for many other reasons, emotional or physical. The object of crying is to attract the attention of her caretaker so that her needs may be met.

In these early years, the response of the adults to the baby's demands will determine how the baby goes about getting her needs met. If the mother responds quickly and consistently to the baby's crying, the infant learns that her needs will be met on demand and as time goes on becomes sure that she will be able to survive. If the baby's needs are met in a caring way (which is not easy at 3:00 a.m. when the other children have been awake all night with croup), then the baby is assured that she will receive both physical support and approval. In other words, the mother and other caretakers approve of her demands and respond to them with love, rather than hostility or resentment.

Now, it will not be all the time that such an idyllic situation occurs. Sometimes Mom, Dad, the kids or Grandfather will be fed up with caring for baby. While they will continue to respond to the basic needs of the infant, they may do so with hostility. If this is an irregular event, the child comes to appreciate that at times some of her legitimate needs will not be met immediately or with smiles, but that generally they will be. Such a child will grow assured of her place within the family and assured of the love of the other members. As she grows older, she learns that when her needs clash with the needs of others, she may not get what she wants. Because it has already been established within the family that it is OK to ask for what you want, the child will not feel threatened by demanding for herself and will continue to do so in the face of disappointments. Failure to get what she wants will result in a display of anger and then perhaps sorrow but will not be accompanied by the fear of loss of love. Her parents have established already that they love the child and that they welcome her demands, even though they may not always grant them.

Now such a child must grow up with a certain attitude towards her own needs and, more particularly, an attitude towards her own power to achieve things that she believes are in her best interests. Her own experience has been that needs she cannot satisfy herself as a child will be treated with love and respect and generally met. Because of this, she believes that it's legitimate to have needs and to ask other people for things. She also has experienced her own ability to get what she wants and needs. As a young baby, she cried and this resulted in people caring for her. She feels powerful. As a young child she asks for what she wants and generally gets it. As an older child she is taught how to do things for herself and how to come for help when she can't manage alone. She grows up believing that she can do things that are in her best interests and that, although at times her interests may clash with others, generally she has the power to benefit herself.

Would this girl grow up with a feeling of control over her own life? And furthermore, would she believe that she could influence the course of her life favorably, either by her own devices or with the assistance of others? I think so. This woman would not feel the need to do things against her interests in order to obtain love and attention. In particular, she would not need to become ill in order to get what she wanted, for she would feel able to get those things directly, either by herself or by asking others. She would feel in control of her own body, knowing that she could keep herself healthy. She would be in no doubt that she could influence her physical state in her favor and with such a belief, would look towards her diet and lifestyle with a view to maintaining her health. Such a person would not allow the environmental hostilities under which we all live to create major illnesses within her body. She has been used to doing things in her best interests and has always believed she has the power to achieve what she wants. Her right to good health she would regard as a matter of course. In other words, this person has no need for illness.

This woman's positivity towards life and her feelings of control over her own destiny will be unconscious. That is, she would be often quite unable to point to any of the psychodynamics we have discussed above. If, however, we listen carefully to this person's language, we will hear the metaphor of a winner. She may say, "I can do that overseas trip next year if I set my mind to it" or, "Last year when we visited India, only two others apart from myself in our party of twenty did not suffer from diarrhea" or "No wonder Jill is ill all the time with a father like that."

She will find herself automatically attracted to like-minded people, namely those who believe in their own capacity to influence their own lives. Most likely she will marry a man who is similarly healthy. Because she was not raised in a family where a child needed to become sick to get attention, she will neither look for a partner who wants to be taken care of nor look for a partner to take care of her. The difference between "taking care of" and "caring for" is important. It is the difference between a belief in non-self-responsibility and self-responsibility. One person may say to another, "I want you to take care of me," meaning, "I want to place responsibility for my life (or this aspect of my life) in your hands." This is the basis of the usual contract drawn up between the public and the medical profession. Another person may say, "I want you to care for me," meaning, "I take responsibility for my own life and within this responsibility I want you to love me."

Now unlike the woman we have been discussing who did not need to hand over responsibility for herself to another because as a child she had been encouraged by her parents to develop a sense of her own strength, let us look at a very common arrangement in Western society to do with illness and being taken care of.

People in Western society are usually aware that a large proportion of their taxes go towards health delivery systems and are generally informed by the media of new technology, new facilities and new costs in the area of health. This concern for our well-being is heightened by exposure to information dealing with environmental pollutants in the air, in food and the water supply, so that it would be a rare person who remained completely impervious to all of this data. Because we dwell upon health matters as a society, we tend to have a good idea of the attitude of potential partners towards their own and others' health. In this climate of concern one may hear a comment such as, "I'd never go out with a smoker" or "If he thinks I'm going to live on the industrial side of town and breathe all that rubbish, he's very mistaken." So we check out the attitudes of our partners with regard to diet, exercise, past illnesses, frequency of time off work, and it is not by chance that a person who often gets ill and wants to be looked after finds and marries a person who likes looking after sick people.

A personal life plan that limits us in some way but which we chose as the best way to get ourselves looked after as kids is called our "script." A man who feels that it is necessary for him to become ill before he can ask for some caring is fulfilling a script decision taken as a child. In this case he limits himself by not simply asking for the caring he wants. For some reason, his parents disapproved of his demands as a child and he became afraid to ask for certain things unless he could show to his parents' satisfaction that his need was legitimate. In his family illness was considered to be a condition warranting caring and he may have needed to use the device of illness to get what he wanted. Hence, the man developed illness whenever he wanted to be cared for and will most likely be living with a partner who shares his belief system and who is more inclined to care for him when he is ill than when he is not.

When people relate to each other in ways which limit both of them they are said to have interlocking scripts. One of the very common interlocking scripts is that of the nurse and the patient. Usually the man is the patient and his wife is the nurse. If he feels unloved, overworked or if the kids are taking up too much of his wife's time, he makes himself ill and she looks after him. If she has been brought up to do this, she will like it and may even encourage illness in her husband. The marriage, revolving around the illness of one member, may go on harmoniously for some time. Then may come a catastrophe. She may get fed up with looking after him and refuse to play the game any longer, in which case he feels hurt and completely unloved and perhaps escalates from a bad back to pneumonia. Or he may decide to not get sick any more because his life is passing by his bedside and she may respond by feeling unwanted and therefore unloved. She may have an affair with a bronchitic down the street. And so it goes until, perhaps, both partners decide they have the responsibility of looking after themselves and their young children and that within this self-responsibility they can both love and be loved.

We began by following the development of a baby growing up in a family where her needs were generally met promptly and with a smile. This baby was allowed to experience her own power to get her needs met and grew into a woman who subconsciously or with partial awareness took charge of her own life and health. What about the other end of the spectrum?

A baby cries and is not fed. A baby is wet and cold and scared and is not changed, made warm and comforted. How do you think this baby's perception of the world will be different? A mother who can't or won't attend to her baby when he cries will be at the other end of the spectrum from one who slavishly attends to baby's every need, even at great personal discomfort, and who may end up smothering the child's independence by needing to shower the baby with love and caring beyond his needs. So here we have two completely opposing attitudes. Both provide the limits to a range of caring for the child, the balanced attitude represented by the woman discussed previously. Let us look at the child whose needs are simply not met.

This unfortunate situation may occur where an unwanted pregnancy, perhaps through ignorance or other factors, is allowed to result in an unwanted baby. If the mother is coerced into keeping the child against her wishes, or is ambivalent about keeping the baby and yet does so, her child may receive minimal basic caring. When the baby cries he is not fed but is allowed to continue crying, often out of earshot of the mother. Or perhaps the mother is busy with a large family and delegates responsibility for feeding the child to other siblings, often the younger ones who are unable to protest as loudly. They get fed up with the baby crying and ignore it. Baby may be offered food when he is not demanding and not offered food when he is. He therefore feels he has little control over his situation as nothing he does to indicate his needs seems to have any bearing on whether or not he is fed. The same situation occurs when he is wet and needs changing or when he is crying because he is scared and needs to be comforted. Nothing he does influences the big people around him. He feels powerless, unable to control his surroundings and in this situation, in order to feel safer and better able to survive in this hostile world, he begins to adapt.

Since he has been unsuccessful in attracting food, warmth and caring from his mother and the family by crying, he may decide that this behavior is not working and start screaming, having tantrums, holding his breath and turning blue, having fits or any other activity devised in desperation to attract the attention he needs. He is fearful that if his needs are not met he will die. Even though the mother and other caretakers may be fully intending to keep him alive, the baby has no experience or evidence of this. The fear is therefore very great and very real. Now if these new behaviors are equally unsuccessful in attracting caring, he may decide that nothing he can do will improve his lot. He stops crying. He becomes very passive and may attract remarks like, "Isn't he a good baby, so calm, he hardly ever seems to cry." This type of experience will lay the basis for a belief in fatalism, that is, the inability to alter the course of one's life. "What will be will be, nothing I can do will make any difference." If people believe they are powerless to influence the course of their own life they will hardly be receptive to the notion that they cause their own illnesses. Rather they will believe that, "You catch colds because other people give you germs" or "The pollutants in the air, foods and water are so bad that you just can't resist them" or "There's cancer in the family so I guess I'll catch it as well." In addition, they will most likely have a high degree of anxiety as a consequence of their early childhood fear about not getting what they want and not surviving, which will raise their adrenalin levels, increase their blood pressure, predispose them to ulcers and colitis and increase their susceptibility to both colds and "accidents." If we believe we are incapable of withstanding these stresses, we sabotage our defense mechanisms and succumb to disease.

If the young boy we have been speaking of cried and was responded to with anger rather than not being responded to at all, then he might have decided that to ask for what he needed was dangerous and that he had better not cry. He may have received love and caring provided he did not kick up a fuss and give

Dad a migraine. The likely outcome of such a situation would be an adult who suppresses his emotions, bottles up anger which he is afraid to express openly, and consequently suffers from any number of physical complaints, hypertension being a likely one. If the personality of the individual refuses to allow the health and legitimate expression of emotion, then disease is practically guaranteed.

We have discussed the girl who, as a consequence of consistently having her needs promptly met, grows up with a faith in her ability to be healthy, and the boy who becomes disease-prone from fatalism and fear. Let us look at what might happen where a child grows up overprotected.

Both Mrs. Jones and her daughter Sally were patients of mine. As the eldest of a family of five children, Mrs. Jones had been given responsibility for looking after some of her younger brothers and sisters from an early age. She had resented these often confining duties, preferring to have fun playing with other children her own age, but her mother was obviously incapable of managing alone, so Mrs. Jones had stayed home and helped out. In the severe winter of 1931, an epidemic of whooping cough had claimed the lives of at least four children in the area, one of whom was her younger sister. Mrs. Jones had felt guilty about her sister's death. It had been her responsibility to keep her sister protected from the cold and despite her mother's reassurances, she had never really forgiven herself.

When Sally was born after three previous pregnancies had all miscarried, Mrs. Jones had naturally been overjoyed. A boy would have been fine, but a girl! She had to be the happiest mother in the world!

When Sally cried, mother was there in an instant,

offering food, changing diapers, cuddling the child and making sure the bed was clean and that no harmful germs could come Sally's way. She found herself rather anxious when strangers wanted to hold or even get close to her child, eventually preferring to have the groceries delivered rather than risk Sally catching a cold by going outside. If a cat or a dog came near the baby she would become really quite frightened, shooing the animal away vigorously. Eventually she noticed that Sally herself would cry whenever an animal or a stranger wanted to be friendly. This she took to be the child's own innate protective mechanisms, confirming her own belief that the situation was unsafe. She really was a devoted mother.

Sally was an excellent scholar, first at school and later at university. Throughout her teenage years she was a loner, disliked boys, disliked going out and generally regarded the world as a scary place. Her health was reasonable but she did seem to catch more than her fair share of colds and trivial ailments, confirming to both herself and her mother that she was delicate. She watched her diet scrupulously, never ate junk food and as a result had beautiful skin and perfect teeth. She looked angelic and was angelic. When she eventually got married and left home, she began suffering recurrent vaginal infections. Her husband agreed to be circumcised as she thought, as did her mother, that this was the cause. The condition did not improve. In addition, she was rarely free of mucus and complained of increasing abdominal upset.

Sally never believed that she was capable of keeping herself healthy. She did not see that she was responsible for being well because the responsibility for her state of health (or anything else for that matter) had never been handed over to her at the appropriate time in childhood. She had been attended to well as a baby but had not grown beyond her dependance on her mother. When her mother was no longer available, she was defenseless, even though she had picked a husband who wanted to take care of her. Sally's unwillingness to take responsibility for herself through fear of the world (as decided upon in childhood) meant she never accepted her own power to be well and as a consequence, she was ill. In this she was not unlike the boy who had not been cared for as a baby and had decided he was powerless to help himself.

The cases we have discussed are not meant to be detailed analyses of often complex family situations. Instead they are intended as simple examples of how early childhood experiences shape the long-term health of the individual. They represent several points along a very broad spectrum.

There are many factors to be considered in examining why people do not take responsibility for their own health, preferring instead to believe that if they become ill they are victims of bad luck. When confronted with the idea that we in fact give ourselves illnesses, many people react with great hostility, pointing to a wide and varied number of examples from their own lives that are intended to prove that illness is beyond the control of the individual. Here we have restricted our examination of this phenomenon to situations where the children never believed they had the power over their own lives and therefore never believed they could prevent illness in themselves.

II

FINDING THE CAUSE

6

The First Contact

The diagnosis and often the treatment of any condition begins at the very first contact between the client and the practitioner. In my case, this is over the telephone, since I make my own appointments. At the conclusion of the usually brief conversation required to effect an appointment, I have roughly assessed the state of health and more importantly, the healing receptivity of the client. The following is a typical call:

"Hello."

"Hello, may I speak with Dr. Harrison please?"

"Yes, this is Dr. Harrison speaking, may I help you?"

"Yes, I'd like to make an appointment to see you."

"Right. It'll mean waiting about two weeks if I haven't seen you before, and you'll be charged the following fees." (An explanation of the exact cost structure and the client's return from insurance follows.)

"Thank you. Actually, I knew the charges already, I've been meaning to come and see you for some time."

"Wednesday, October 5, at 4:00 p.m.? The consultation will last for an hour."

"Thank you, Doctor, I'll see you then.

My information so far is that I'm dealing with a well-educated middle-aged woman, who has taken a decision to come and see me from a position of some power and self-responsibility. She has not come immediately but waited some months before making the appointment, and I therefore know she puts safety first but is prepared to risk when necessary. No doubt she knows a lot about my treatment from talking with the friends who recommended me. More information about how far she's prepared to take the notion that we give ourselves illness will have to wait until the actual appointment. I know also from the telephone conversation that she has already decided that she's prepared to take responsibility for the financial burden of the appointment. This information has come from the content of our conversation. The tone of voice is equally, if not more, important.

If she sounds angry, I differentiate between anger directed at me or at others. This tells me if I'm dealing with someone who is angry that her professional caretakers, usually the medical profession, have not solved her problem. In these circumstances, I can anticipate the client setting me up to be yet another useless professional who fails to help her. This is valuable information that, if not recognized, can mean a considerable waste of time.

Or the client may have a helpless, breathless voice that is saying, "I cannot look after myself. If I ap-

pear helpless enough surely someone will assist me."
And of course most doctors love to be helpers and
many will go along with the client and say, "Yes, what
rotten luck you're suffering from cancer, let me help
you." After the rescuing doctor has been well and
truly entangled in his and the client's mutually laid
net, the client will often, as her condition worsens, ac-
cuse the doctor of being hopeless, uncaring or of being
a false prophet. The doctor in turn becomes angry at
being abused for his efforts and says that the client
"doesn't want to get well anyway!" Both end up feeling
bad because neither has been prepared to admit that
the client made herself ill. The doctor, for his part, is
scared that unless he maintains the illusion of fate as
the cause of the disease and unless he can be helpful,
he is redundant. It is also dangerous for him to acknowledge the role the client plays in her own illness,
because logically that proportion the client admits as
"self-caused" will then become available for "self-
cure." This he sees as threatening to his livelihood.

Consider the following telephone conversation:

"Hello."

"Hello, may I speak with Dr. Harrison
please?"

"Yes, Dr. Harrison speaking, may I help
you?"

"Yes, I'm calling to make an appointment for
my husband—he's at work right now."

"I'm not prepared to make an appointment
for him through another person. If your husband wants to see me, he'll have to call
himself."

"I see, well thank you, I'll tell him."

"You're welcome, goodbye."

Finding the Cause

Except in the case of the diminished responsibility of childhood, making appointments for relatives is a game, and to accept the appointment will generally involve the doctor in a situation that uses the illness of one partner for the benefit of both. If the patient calls up later, then I have gained some valuable information, and if his nose is put out of joint to such an extent that he doesn't call, then I have saved myself the trouble of spending an hour with someone who wasn't ready to look at himself. Later he may feel safe to do so.

At first contact, clients will commonly attempt to assess whether a doctor will be an ally in their persecution of the orthodox medical profession. This is tantamount to establishing that the doctor agrees that they are not responsible for their own illness.

"Hello."

"Hello, may I speak with Dr. Harrison please?"

"Speaking."

"Oh, Doctor, I'm so glad I reached you, I've been trying for a couple of weeks now and you never seem to be there." (The content is condemnatory despite a friendly, effusive, and somewhat seductive mood.)

"I've been here all along, how can I help you?"

"Well, I suffer terribly from arthritis and my local doctor said there was nothing more he could do. All he does is give me more and more drugs. Even the specialist reckoned I'd be in a wheelchair by the time I'm sixty and I hate being a burden on people, especially my poor old hubby who's under the doctor's care himself. We're on Social Security you know, nobody cares about us, the cost of living is so high, you can't afford fresh vegetables even. . .

I interrupt, "You may know from the person who recommended me, in cases such as yours I believe diet plays a large part, and the likelihood is that yours will be changed substantially."

"Doctor, we eat very well given our meager means, and . . . "

"I can't discuss this over the telephone. You might consider whether you're prepared to undergo a long and significant dietary prescription, and if you decide you are, then I'll be pleased to make an appointment for you." (My tone indicates the end of the conversation.)

"Very well, Doctor, thank you!"

"You're welcome."

This caller may decide that the initial contact was encouraging and come and see me. Having trotted out the usual helpless game and got nowhere with it, she may decide I'm capable of helping her after all. In that case, she may do quite well in therapy, and while substantially altering her diet, I will engage her in an examination of the advantages in her being ill. She has already indicated that her husband is significant, and my guess is that they are playing "I'm sicker than you are." If she doesn't come along, I assume that what I was offering was unattractive and that she will continue as she is until the symptoms worsen or she's prepared to risk more. Either way, I have learned something of value in our exchange and perhaps she has as well.

Many telephone conversations will be longer than the ones reported but whatever the length or complexity, I follow some basic principles. I take the view that there's a component of the disease, small or large, that's a consequence of the client's own actions. I indicate that this is a good thing as that part of the illness is available for them to cure. I avoid the words blame and fault. I avoid clients who want to fight if I see that my chances of winning are slight. Sometimes I recommend them to other practitioners who I think can help them. I avoid claiming a mortgage on the truth. I am generally enthusiastic about their prospects. I make good use of the anger, sorrows, frustrations and resentments directed towards people who are supposed to heal them. I never let the client hand me the burden of responsibility for her own illness. This all takes place during the initial telephone conversation, and when I first see the client, I recall what she previously said.

The actual appointment time settled on by the client is also significant. A business person who interrupts a busy schedule to attend has decided that she needs to do something about her condition even if her day is disrupted. People who argue about the fact that I don't see people out of hours will still be at the stage of believing that, as they are the victims of illness, it's unreasonable for them to be inconvenienced by it. Barriers put in the way of people getting what they want can be prudently used to assess the form of therapy that will be most effective for them. I am reminded of an American colleague who would not make appointments for specific times within the day. His clients arrived at 9:00 a.m. and might not be seen until 5:00 p.m. The receptionist arranged activities such as nutrition and anti-smoking films, and in fine weather, walks. By the time they were seen by the doctor, they often had a new perspective on their illness. He argued that as he didn't know what he would be dealing with until he began investigating it, the time required might vary from ten minutes to three hours. My "hurry up" driver would find such an arrangement intolerable!

THE FIRST ATTENDANCE

One of the advantages of not having a large staff and greeting my patients personally in the waiting room is that I see the client before she actually enters my office. By that time, she has already modified her behavior significantly, especially if she has a long history of attending medical practitioners. She feels she's expected to behave in a certain way. This will often be fostered by the doctor and almost always by the medical receptionist.

The game of "You are privileged to be able to see me," which maintains the patient in a one-down position, keeps the practitioner divorced from the real problem and, most importantly, aims at keeping the patient feeling guilty about being ill and taking up everyone's valuable time, usually begins with the medical receptionist. For this purpose the receptionist is often abrupt, depersonalized and a very hard person to reason with if she's taken it upon herself or has been instructed to protect the doctor from the public. In addition, the mood of the client has often altered a great deal by having to run this gauntlet in the reasonable attempt to consult the doctor. This may interfere with the diagnosis.

In sorting out why a child has at this time given himself earache, it's invaluable to hear Mother or Father herding him, along with the other children, into the office. If both parents attend the consultation, which I encourage, it's even better.

"Mom, if the doctor says I'm all right, can I have a chocolate fudge afterwards?"

"No, you cannot!"

"But Mom, when Barnie went to the doctor last time you bought him one."

"Yes, but he was sick, the doctor said his ears were very bad."

"Gee, Mom, that's not fair."

"Be quiet, here's the doctor to see you."

The message from Mom to young Johnny here is quite clear. If you want a chocoloate fudge, then you have to earn it, and you do that by being very sick. This rewards illness and penalizes wellness, and believe it or not, is by far the most common way in which families act. It directly descends from the notion that people who get ill have little say in the matter, and are simply the victims of circumstance. Therefore, when they fall ill and are "brave," they are rewarded. You can be very sure that if Johnny's ears aren't bad enough this time to earn a chocolate fudge, they will be next time.

A family with three children have consulted me since the girl was born. The elder boy was five, and had suffered many complaints, all of them minor. The girl, who was three, had been exceptionally well, much to her irritation at times. When she came into the office, I was sure to listen to her chest and look into her ears. She found the attention very exciting, even though there was nothing wrong with her. On these occasions her brother was the patient. The one-year-old boy had been well and, given the very much more relaxed style of child-rearing in the family that came with experience, I expect he always will be. He was told that the world was safe, that he could expect to be well, and that there was no need to make himself ill.

One evening, while the three children were playing at home in the living room, both parents overheard the elder boy say to his sister, "If you want Mommy to look after you, just get sick, that's what I do!" Remember, this is a five-year-old patient telling his three-year-old sister how to get cared for. When I was told this story by his mother, I was amazed at the boy's command of the family psychodynamics. It's a mistake to believe that children don't understand what happens in families. They understand very well, and since their energies in the matter are directed solely towards being cared for, their perceptions are usually very accurate. Also, because they aren't yet conditioned into secrecy and shame, they'll tell you what's happening, if you ask them. In the case of this young boy, the parents and I now reward him when he's well and not when he's ill. Eventually, when he believes that he'll be cared for without being ill, which was the old pattern, he'll start to be well. The body will also need time to recover from the damage caused by organisms made dangerous by a physiology not directed towards keeping itself healthy.

Now all of this essential information may be lost by not being within earshot when the family is interacting as they come through the door of the building. Until they know you, children will be subdued in the presence of the doctor, especially if under parental pressure. Parents in turn often feel very guilty when their children are ill, and if this isn't dealt with, the children's chances of resolving the need to be ill are reduced.

With children, the next information comes from watching them play with the toys in the waiting room. I often bring the toys into the office so that I can observe them at play while I'm getting the details from the parents. This will usually tell me the pecking order of the family, who chastises who when the younger child has a toy pulled away from him and begins to cry, and what behavior has proven effective in the past for attracting parental attention. Where children have been born within two years of each other, I observe the older one's attitude towards the younger. One of the most common illness dynamics in families is the older of two children of similar ages getting ill for attention. It makes sense. The secure world of the elder child is shattered by the arrival of the new baby, and any behavior that results in his receiving more attention will be repeated. There will often be an exaggerated caring for the younger sibling by the elder child. When mother's attention is diverted, the elder child may twist the younger's arm. I wonder whether I'm becoming too cynical when I say that I distrust children caring for those in the family who are only slightly younger than themselves. Such a caring attitude is, of course, much praised and paraded in front of relatives and neighbors but as new babies are rarely in the best interests of slightly older siblings, I suspect the older children unconsciously want to harm the baby. That would be natural.

Adults are just as informative as children, often while trying hard not to be. Usually they have their behavior more under control and the practitioner must be very observant if he wants to find out the real problem. I believe there's a place for shoe therapists, hat therapists, clothes, car, ring and perfume therapists. Each of these accouterments and many others tell you with whom you're dealing. What's being said may be of secondary importance.

The choice of chair is significant. In the waiting room I have several quite different styles of chair.

They face different directions and are close to either the books, the plants or the door. Some can be seen readily as I emerge from the office, others are well hidden from direct view. The chair the client chooses will be as specific as his choice of clothing and will reflect his prevailing mood.

THE GENERAL APPEARANCE

One of the moments of truth in the process of preliminary diagnosis occurs when the client and the practitioner come face to face for the first time. The look on the client's face may vary from "This was a good idea, I like the look of this guy," to "Just my luck, I've struck some sort of hippie!" There may also be pleasure, fear, excitement, amusement, indifference or anger (particularly if I remind them of someone who is a significant figure in their lives).

In turn, the immediate impression that the client makes upon me is lasting. The first whole body image, or Gestalt, will be an accurate reflection of her most cherished dreams, her greatest disappointments, the way she views herself, her illness and the world. I see stored-up anger in the flushed face and the red margins of the eyes. The stooped walk and the hunched shoulders show the fear that leads to poor kidney function and ear infections, and in the bridge of the nose the chronic allergy and sinus sufferer reveals her sorrow.

I'm aware of the despair of the chronically ill, or the smugness of the multiple sclerosis sufferer who has achieved the incapacity she wanted. I see the fear of anticipating the long haul back to health, and the anger of being confronted by yet another healing professional. Fear, anger, joy and sorrow are there for all to see. We can all see in others' faces a pictorial history of their lives. There's no hiding, no editing, no mask, for how can a person alter the way she looks? The very attempt is obvious, and reflects exactly what she's feeling and thinking at the time. Every line tells of a past experience either satisfactorily resolved or hidden away at the back of the mind where it continues to smolder.

DIAGNOSIS BY THE FACE—PHYSIOGNOMY

The set of the mouth is vital in establishing why the client has made herself ill. Forced emotions are easily detected, such as the thinning of the corners of the mouth in clients who smile their way through a tragic history, or the clenched-teeth smile of the chronically angry. With the latter no stethoscope is needed, for the diagnosis of hypertension is obvious. The size of the upper lip often reflects the emotional flexibility of the client. A large, full, mobile upper lip is indicative of someone who has smiled a lot from the joys of childhood. Suppression of any emotions results in a thinner upper lip. One must allow for the genetic element, of course, but I've seen these things change in therapy, and in people in their forties. Pouting, that occurs when people are dissatisfied with what they have, but are afraid to get what they want, expresses itself in a large protuberant lower lip. This state of chronic sadness and fear will eventually result in internal changes in the body, just as it caused a large lip. If I exercise my biceps for any reason I'll end up with large biceps. If the facial and lip muscles are repeatedly used to express certain emotions, those emotions will eventually be visible in the face. Similarly, the internal organs will be altered by the chronic stresses of predominant emotions, particularly if those emotions are not expressed but internalized. It is of old emotions that haven't been expressed and forgotten, but have been retained through fear, that disease is made. Expressing thoughts and feelings as they occur allows the body to return to a state of resting balance. In such cases the face becomes lively and flexible, expressing a myriad expressions.

Chronic anger, that is prevalent in those multicultural societies where people struggle to live in harmony together, manifests itself in the structure of the jawline. The powerful chewing muscles at the angle of the jaw enlarge in cases where it was not safe to yell at parents. In these circumstances, particularly if the individual was expected to smile instead, she will learn to smile through clenched teeth. When she gets angry, she won't open her mouth wide and yell but separate her lips and keep her teeth together instead. She tends to snarl rather than be openly angry. Such a person will often end up getting what she wants indirectly, and in a manner that rarely satisfies her and often leaves others with whom she interacts feeling uncomfortable. When one yells through clenched teeth, the anger may be regarded as bouncing off the back of the teeth and going back deep down inside, from whence it continues to cause further havoc. To release the muscle tension associated with anger, it's necessary to open the mouth wide and stretch the jaw muscles. The pupils dilate, the adrenalin level increases and the blood pressure rises. When the anger is fully dealt with, all of these physiological reactions return to normal. If someone buries her anger, the blood pressure remains higher longer and eventually becomes chronically elevated. This is hypertension. In addition, the liver (the seat of anger, so the Chinese have claimed for three-thousand years) will be healthy if anger is expressed. If the liver is functioning well, the eyes will be clear and bright. According to the theory of macrobiotics, general health is reflected in the position of the iris within the eye socket. The more white showing beneath the iris, the worse the state of health.

The eyes are also invaluable in determining how scared the client is. Chronic fear will result (once again according to the Chinese) in a disturbance of kidney function, that in turn causes puffiness and often a blue discoloration about the eyes. We've all experienced the urinary frequency associated with fear before exams or a sporting contest. Sometimes the eyes will be red and the eyelid margins will be both red and swollen. When I see this, I wonder if the client needs to cry, and for some reason has been stopping herself. If she's been suppressing other emotions as well, then the odds are she'll be depressed, and I'll expect her to tell me later that she's suffering from either sinusitis or constipation, or more commonly both. Embryologically (embryology is that branch of science concerned with the development of the body), the skin and the brain come from the same basic tissue called "ectoderm." Because of this early common origin, the skin reflects our emotional state quickly and accurately. Within the practice of dermatology (diseases of the skin), a large number of conditions are recognized as being of a psychological origin (psychogenic). The skin of the face shows both chronic emotions and acute ones, such as blushing. The precise texture of the skin may be difficult to see at first, and may have to await the formal examination, expecially if make-up is used. However, the general impression of the skin as a significant part of the personality will be obvious. If the skin is either perfect, on the one hand, or suffering from acne, dermatitis, psoriasis or excessive oil on the other, you can be sure that it's important to the client's body image. If clients haven't liked themselves much in the past, they'll often advertise the fact in their face. By such a mechanism they reaffirm the world as a lousy place, informing people of their suffering indirectly while often openly denying it, and making sure they never face their real fears. "If only I had good skin!" or "Why me?" People with skin that is blemish-free will often be suffering other more serious ailments, but "soldiering on bravely." They may have a need to appear perfect to the world, although suffering both mentally and physically in private. I've found intestinal problems to be common in this group. The skin at the side of the nose is often scaly and inflamed in chronic fear and sadness, and if it is, I'll take more time during the formal examination of the ears, as often the skin will be similarly affected in the external ear canal. The general skin texture is noted for color and general vitality, but this is within the realm of orthodox diagnosis and much has been made of it elsewhere. My concern is to use the facial anatomy to diagnose the emotional state and from there the physiological disturbance that follows (or vice versa). This is called physiognomy.

BODY SHAPE AND SEXUALITY

I will next be attracted to other outstanding features of the client's body and clothing. My attention will be drawn to those areas she has highlighted, either wittingly or unwittingly, and in both cases these will be features that are of significance to the person herself. In addition, my own personal bias will affect the areas of the body that I look at first. My diagnostic abilities are compatible with my personality, so that I pick up some things easily and miss others completely. Those things that are important, but which I habitually ignore, will result in my handling some cases poorly and those people will eventually stop coming to see me. This is inevitable.

I take great note of general body shape. Within the category of body shape or habitus I include the person's attitude to her own sexuality. The individual may appear to me as a gazelle, a cat, a proud lion, a bird, a hippopotamus, a field mouse or a sloth. Clients may stand erect, men with their pelvis inclined slightly forward inviting an appreciation of their genitals, and with their neck and shoulders broad, relaxed and powerful. Women may project their breasts forward in sexual display and walk with both grace and fluidity, their more mobile pelvis swaying gently as they enjoy their own body. Where there's been a childhood direction to ignore feelings but where either or both parents were comfortable with their sexuality, there may be an exaggeration of the client's sexuality at the expense of expressing sadness, fear and anger. She may be at ease with multiple casual relationships but uncomfortable with genuine closeness. In such cases the woman may have make-up that is overdone and scarcely concealed breasts. She may rush into premature intimacy. Men overdisplaying their sexuality will have a certain swagger to their walk and a dress sense that is more flamboyant than attractive. On the other hand, men who continually turn up to appointments in clothing that is drab and shapeless and when undressed reveal a trim, attractive, male physique, are obviously suppressing their sexuality.

Between the over- and underdressing is a set of clothes for men that are functional and comfortable, which show their masculinity to advantage and which give an indication that they are sexually potent. Women will be similarly attired with what they consider their best features highlighted. Teenage girls who are embarrassed by their breasts often walk with a stoop to conceal them, or hunch their shoulders if they don't want to lose height. Boys testing their fledgling sexuality will make sure their clothing conceals their penis, so that they can both avoid the embarrassment and enjoy the thrill of an erection. Even younger children's clothing will reflect the attitudes of their parents, usually the mother. Young girls in particular learn very early that they are sexually attractive to men, and it's common to have a two-year-old flaunting her body in front of men in a manner usually reserved for B-grade movies. In a child this can be very attractive, and if the habit is encouraged it will last into adulthood.

Suppression or overuse of any bodily system will result in imbalance. If this goes on long enough, exhaustion and disease result. People who either suppress their sexuality or abuse it will eventually complain of a disease of the sexual organs: the penis and testicles in men; or breasts, ovaries, tubes, womb and vaginal area in women. Sexual history will be part of the later more detailed client history, as will a sexual examination, but at this point of first contact much of this information is available to the astute observer. General appearance will reflect the later sexual history. Where the appearance and the story conflict, then I question the story.

Sexuality aside, the general body shape is equally revealing in other ways. If people stand or walk hunched over and are shabbily dressed, it's reasonable to assume that at the time they regard themselves as shabby, unless they have dressed intending to mislead you, which happens sometimes and will be evident elsewhere. Depression reveals itself in the clothing and the walk; the voice is powerless. Anger will often produce a tight, muscular body with little fluidity, often the shape of professional sports persons; while sadness is evident in stooped shoulders and irregular breathing. Someone who is afraid will rarely look at you directly, often has darting eye movements as if looking for danger, and breathes in a shallow, rapid manner.

We all have the ability to see these things in others. We do it ourselves every day to avoid situations that we don't want to confront. The avoidance behavior is automatic. It's unnecessary to be conscious of those individual features we are monitoring. We just know that right now there's something about another person that makes us uncomfortable and we want to stay away from her.

Diagnostically, however, to overlook the various physical reflections of the underlying psychological states is to ignore the most valuable source of unedited information. A person who stands up straight every day of her life appears quite different to one who normally walks bent over, but has straightened for the occasion. You can tell this by simply looking at her. Dialogue needn't cloud the matter. An appreciation of the psychological state begins at the point of first contact and is essential if anything beyond a cursory and superficial consultation is intended. Treatment without this information would be like trying to repair a broken-down car by painting it.

The color, texture, style and grooming of the hair will provide information on a client's feelings now, and in the recent and distant past. Premature graying or balding may indicate chronic tension and underlying high blood pressure. Dry, lifeless hair, as described in televison advertisements, may reflect a similar state of mind. A friend of mine calls such hair "frayed nerve ends." Grooming of the hair is as helpful as clothing in establishing a person's self-image. Hair has long been used in our society to indicate an individual's social and political status. The pop culture, hippies, street gangs, Eastern religious sects, punk rockers, the business fraternity and politicians have all used hairstyles to advertise their allegiances. There's obviously a strong genetic element to hair distribution, color and texture but nevertheless, it's still a valuable display, particularly as it can be changed quite radically, unlike the face, in a short time.

In our society, certain appearances are associated with wealth or poverty. People can therefore dress to appear as if they do or don't have money. If a person who is quite wealthy or has worked hard to improve her financial position continues to dress as though she is still poor or perhaps a student, that's significant. She'll often want to be seen as a loser and still regard herself as such. To acknowledge that she's "made it" would arouse in her the fear of contradicting a parent who told her she'd fail. Becoming successful threatens the parental attribution, for the parent message is interpreted by the child as being, "I'll only love you as long as you don't make it" or often, "I'll only love you if you don't do better than I." Such an individual will often be suffering from a complaint that won't kill her, but will prevent her from achieving her full potential in her chosen occupation. Arthritis is an example. "If I didn't have arthritis I reckon I'd have been a better lawyer than Dad. It's so debilitating. . ."

When I meet a client face to face for the first time, I'm careful to note the tone and the exact content of her greeting. The actual words used in this and in any interchange come unedited from her subconscious and more often than not are a true reflection of what she means, as opposed to a hasty alteration. "Hello, Mr., I mean Dr. Harrison" may indicate a hopeless player— "Help me because I'm incompetent," or a rebellious nature—"Don't put on your doctor's airs with me!" The first person may be using her illness as a way of being cared for, while the second has not forgiven her parents and may be making herself sick to stay angry with them. If she stays sick enough, long enough, then surely they'll change and love her as she wants (even though they may have died years ago). Without resolution of these underlying psychodynamics, true cure of the disease is not possible.

THE VOICE

Hostility, fear, sadness and joy are always evident in the voice. There's a certain resonance to a happy person's voice. There is no inflammation of the sinuses and this means the voice box gives the voice a mellow, powerful quality. In addition, the vocal cords are healthy, suffering neither from abuse nor inflammation. The airstream delivered by the lungs to the vocal cords is steady and strong. The lips and the facial muscles that help to shape the airstream are flexible and the facial expression and the quality of the voice are synchronized. There's a wide range of vocal abilities, reflecting the person's ability to express what she's feeling at the time. A happy person will be able and willing to sing.

A person who suppresses her anger usually speaks with her mouth partially closed, for fear of exposing her wrath. The small mouth aperture and the limited range of movement of the upper lip, causes the voice to sound "thin." The upper lip in these people is narrow from lack of exercise, as in the abandonment of laughter, and from being continually drawn into a contrived smile. The final shaping of the airstream is therefore affected. The airstream is less steady because there's a permanent battle between the client's angry little kid who wants to scream, and her controlling grown-up. The result is a variable delivery of air to vocal cords already stretched tight by muscular tension. A harsh abrasive voice caused by the vocal cords hitting each other may result. This is called "vocal attack."

Where sadness predominates, the voice will be weak and often breathless. The mouth and vocal cords "wave in the breeze," resulting in a voice with a lack of impact and conviction. The air delivery will reflect indecision about whether to breathe or not, especially in severe depression, and sometimes sighing will be a feature as will speaking while inhaling. A wavering of the voice and a quiver of the bottom lip may be observed in someone struggling not to cry. If crying has been suppressed, there may be chronic inflammation of the sinuses with a muffling of the vocal resonance. The voice may have a nasal quality caused by the chronically swollen lining of the nose and the resultant partially obstructed airway.

I am listening for two levels of feelings: the immediate (or spontaneous) and the past (or "racket"). We all recognize the former easily, but the latter are often more subtle and, although we register them accurately, we may not be consciously aware of them. As "racket feelings" are active over a long period of time, they affect the voice, body musculature and internal organs profoundly, and are therefore diagnostically invaluable.

Finding the Cause

Fear is probably the most common racket feeling. A racket feeling is a common feeling emanating from unresolved childhood conflicts. The feeling may appear to come from the "here and now," but is really a revival of old emotions that are simply triggered by the immediate situation. A man who repeatedly assaults people for no apparent reason, and whose father beat him as a child, is probably still very angry from childhood. The anger is left over. If people are depressed all the time, it's not because they have nothing to be positive about but because they are "racket sad." The sadness comes from their childhood. If they're angry all the time, it's because they are "racket angry," not because they're singled out by fate to have bad luck. Some individuals are "racket happy." They go around with a smile on their faces while hurting inside. "Racket fear" underlies most racket feelings. The large majority of people in Western society have a degree of this fear. It is the most basic of all the racket feelings, as it's really the fear of not surviving as a child. This fear results in various adaptations. If there was doubt in the mind of either parent that they had the resources or the inclination to keep a child alive, or their mood reflected a general societal anxiety with the state of the world (caused, for example, by the Cold War of the 1950s or the Vietnam War of the 1960s), doubt may have entered the child's mind as to whether she could survive this danger. This doubt may have been negated by a greater preponderance of positive messages and simply be present in traces, or may dominate a person's feeling, thinking and behavior. Either way, it remains very obvious in the face and voice. Being scared is the most significant precursor to illness that I know.

The diagram on p. 113 indicates a common arrangement of racket anger, sadness and joy as they are

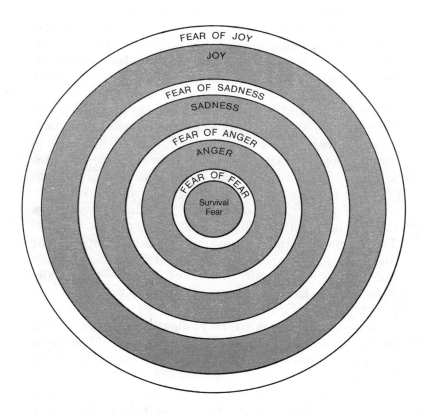

A common arrangement of the "racquet feelings" (shaded area)
as they have been used to protect an individual from confronting his
fear of survival.

used to protect an individual from confronting his basic racket feeling, the fear of not surviving. Between each racket feeling is a layer of fear, an emotion used by the individual to discourage his awareness of the structure of his defenses. All layers may be associated with their own physical signs and symptoms, accounting for changes in the nature of the client's complaints as therapy proceeds.

The opposite to a racket feeling is one that arises spontaneously and is fully expressed so that none of it remains from that particular stimulus. If someone is clumsy and nearly runs you over in his car, you scream, "Hey, watch what you're damn well doing!" You feel mad as hell for a minute or two and then it's gone. If your lover leaves you for another, you cry every night for a month and then you're over it. There's no residual sadness left, so that when the cat dies, you don't cry for weeks or get depressed, which for most people would be racket sadness, caused by suppressing their sadness at their lover's defection and not the cat's death.

Beyond the fear is joy. Happiness is not the opposite of fear, anger or sadness. Happiness is an absence of racket (or leftover) feelings, and a preparedness to spontaneously feel joy, anger, sadness and fear.

The voice of a person who's chronically afraid, which is a racket feeling, will be wavering, apparently struggling against great odds to even be heard, and the speech may begin and end abruptly. The breathing will be shallow and rapid, with little expansion of the chest wall. A feature of scared people is that they hunch their shoulders to hide their chest from view, as the heart is considered vulnerable. This further restricts the delivery of air to the vocal cords, whose movements already reflect the general indecision of the body musculature. These people don't trust life.

They certainly don't trust themselves to stay well.

Both levels of feelings, the spontaneous and the racket, will be evident in the face, general body shape, and the voice. Racket feelings will be etched into the face by time. Immediate or spontaneous emotion will overlie the general contour of the face, so that a generally happy person with a flexible and expressive face may show the grief caused by the recent loss of a loved one. Similarly, an individual who has generally cared for her appearance may appear slightly ruffled on the day I see her. The racket feelings are of great importance in diagnosing the basis of an individual's illness. Because such feelings have been active for a long time, the external, visible changes will indicate alterations to the physiology and later the anatomy of the internal organs. As they may not yet have produced symptoms, a diagnosis of the psychological state can be predictive and therefore preventive.

Till now, there's been no need to take much notice of the *content* of the client's conversation. That will be important later, but right now the important thing is to observe her so that an independent impression of her problem may begin to take shape. I assume that if clients were so objective about themselves that they could see their way clearly, they would not have consulted me in the first place. Therefore it's of real value to allow an intuitive impression, based on subtle observation, to affect the practitioner. This is how fortune-tellers, tarot-card readers, palmists and most astrologers work. It's not what clients are saying but how they are saying it, not how they are trying to appear but how they look.

In addition, it's essential for the doctor to know something of herself. If she finds angry men sexy and she's feeling sexy, then she's probably dealing with an angry man. The practitioner needs to witness her own internal processes and seek confirmation of her observations at a later point. The fact that doctors and therapists have their own problems does not prevent them from being aware of what is happening with clients. In fact, they are usually interested in why others make *themselves* ill because they (the doctors) make themselves ill. Therapists who are motivated to resolve their own problems can be of help to clients wishing to help themselves.

After introducing myself to a client in the waiting room, some light conversation usually follows as I lead the way to the surgery proper, or office as I prefer to call it. I listen to what he's saying carefully during this time, because he's often off-guard. He may notice paintings, or comment on the color of the walls, or look straight ahead in an effort not to notice anything. Everything he does is used to assemble and evolve a picture of who he is and why he is making himself ill. It's impossible for him not to react. Even not reacting is a reaction.

By the time the client and I sit down at the desk for the formal history, I could write a chapter of a book about him. Very often I can name the illness he will complain of before he tells me. It's not some magic or some special power I possess, but simple observation based on the premise that the disease the client suffers from is an integral part of his personality, and that personality is observable.

All of this has taken no more than one minute. I'm now ready for the next step, the history of the illness or, to my mind, the history of the client's physiological response to life thus far.

7

History and Examination

WHAT IS THE PROBLEM

It is now the client's turn. I listen to what the client is saying about his illness and once again, how he is saying it. I give him the opportunity to tell me in his own words and at his own speed what he thinks is wrong with him, and where he feels that he's made mistakes in the management of his own health. I don't lead him in the early stages, as it is his opinion of his problem that's important, not a medical label that I, through expediency or convenience, may need to tag him with. By resisting the temptation to categorize him as suffering from an orthodox disease, which in reality bears little resemblance to his actual complaint, I am rewarded by a fascinating insight into the relationship between his bodily dysfunction and the mind that spawned and nurtured it.

If nerve pain of the lower limb in a woman with business problems is sciatica, then what is nerve pain in the lower limb of a man who has just chosen to leave his family? Surely not sciatica! The two presenting symptoms are the same or similar but the cause (pathogenesis) and therefore the treatment is entirely different. Standardized inflexible treatments follow the expedient labeling of discomforts, needs, wants, frustrations, aspirations, fears and destinies, as being certain diseases. Dis-eases they are, but the same they are not.

I then ask the client a series of questions in order to elicit which systems of the body he has chosen to fulfill his need for an illness at this time, and how dysfunctional he has made those systems. This is known as the systems analysis, which is outlined on pages 122-131.

By following a standardized format here, I'm able to give examples of commonly suffered illnesses as they relate to the psychological profile (see Chapter 11) of the sufferers. As you read this section, you will begin to understand your own role in conditions from which you have been suffering. You now have two equally valid general options: to continue with the illness or to remove it.

After the client has been given the opportunity to include all the information that he thinks necessary, I run through the following checklist in my mind, asking some of the questions and eliminating others. As you will see in the interpretations of this data that immediately follows, I continually address myself to the client's motives for being ill or well, and my enquiry will reflect leads that I intuitively follow up and tangents that I think warrant exploration.

A physical examination follows:

Personal Details

Title:
Name:

Age:
Date of birth:
Address:
Telephone no:
Number of children:

The Presenting Complaints

The major complaint.
What parts are affected?
How severe is it?
How long have you had it?
Describe a typical attack.
How frequent are the attacks?
Are they becoming more or less frequent?
Are they becoming more or less severe?
What other parts of the body are affected by this
     problem?
Is there any pain?
How severe is the pain?
Where is the pain?
When is the pain a problem?
Is the pain associated with any other malfunction?
Does the pain radiate to other areas?
What is the nature of the pain? (sharp, dull throb-
     bing, colic, etc.)
Do you feel nauseous?
Do you vomit?
What investigations have you already had?
Who have you seen before about this complaint?
What was their diagnosis?
What laboratory tests have you had?
Have you had surgery for this complaint?
Have you had any previous treatments for this con-
     dition?

Are you having treatment at present?
What, and by whom?
Previous drug treatments—have you had any?
Current medications?
Drugs?
Herbal treatments?
Vitamins?
What connections do you make between this illness
    and your mental state, if any?
What do you think is your problem?
What do you want to do about it?
Have you any general comments you would like to
    make about the illness or yourself?
What has been happening in your life recently?

Complaint no. 2
Complaint no. 3
Complaint no. 4
Complaint no. 5
Etcetera

(The same questions are asked about every complaint the client lists, and they are encouraged to
list everything. The more information gained about
the body's reaction to the psychological state and
vice versa, the more accurate the diagnosis.)

The Past History

What operations have you had?
What was the diagnosis on those occasions?
When were the operations performed?
By whom were they performed?

(In contemporary medical practice it is no longer a

logical assumption that if an operation has been performed then it was for a good reason, a correct diagnosis or necessarily in the patient's interest.)

What serious medical illnesses have you had?
When, and what were they?
What treatment did you have at the time?
Are you still having treatment for these?
What is that treatment?

What childhood illnesses did you have?
Were you sick as a child? (This question checks the reality of the previous question against the body image of either being well or sickly.)

Have you ever had hepatitis, epilepsy, asthma, eczema, rheumatic fever, glandular fever?
When, and how severely?
How long did you take to recover?

The Family History

Is there a family history of any illness?
Did any of your family suffer from the same complaint as you?
Are your parents alive?
Are your children alive and well?
Is there any illness with the following family members that is significant to you?
Mother
Father
Grandparents
Aunts
Uncles
Siblings

Finding the Cause

Children

Is there any other person that you consider influenced the course of your disease?

Are your siblings well?

If they are ill, what are their complaints?

Compare your body shape with that of your siblings.

Compare your body shape with that of your children.

Compare your general state of health with your siblings, parents, children.

List the names and ages of your siblings and your children.

Who in your family as a child was "always ill?"

Who in your family as a child was "always well?"

Can you recall what was said in your family as a child about you being ill and about you being well?

Were there any general complaints made when you were a child about illness, wellness and people who were "always ill" or "always well?"

Do you make comments about people being ill or well?

What are they, and about whom do you make them?

The Systems Analysis

Gastro-Intestinal System

Hop on the scales and I'll weigh you.

Has your weight increased, decreased or remained steady?

Over what period of time has it increased or decreased?

How do you rate your appetite?
How often do you eat, and at what times?
How much do you eat?

Tell me about your bowels.
How many times a day do you use them?
What is the consistency of your bowel motion? Is it
    long and pointed, firmer or softer than that? Is
    it formed at all? Is it loose? Does it vary?
Is there any blood in your bowel motion?
When?
How much?
Bright or dark?
What is the color of your bowel motion?
Does the color ever change?
Do your feces float or sink in the toilet?
Is there any undigested material present in your
    bowel motions?
Is there any pain when you use your bowels?
How does the variation in your bowels correspond to
    what is happening in your life at the time?
Do you know at what age you were toilet trained?
Are you willing to defecate in front of family,
    friends or strangers?
Do you squat or sit on the toilet?
By what method do you clean your anus following
    defecation?
How is your bowel function related to your current
    complaints?

Have you any abdominal pain?
    (If yes, repeat the pain questions from the
    presenting complaint.)
Do you suffer from epigastric pain (heartburn)?
How is that related to meals?

Finding the Cause

How long after a meal do you feel the pain?
Put one finger on where it is?
How long does it last?
What do you take to relieve it?
Is it worse in any position? (lying down or bending
    over)
Do you feel nauseous or vomit?
To what events in your life is it related?
Do you suffer from hemorrhoids?
How long have you had them?
What makes them better?
What makes them worse?
Do you have them now?

The Respiratory System

Do you smoke?
What do you smoke?
Cigarettes, a pipe, marijuana?
How many do you smoke and at what times?
For how long have you been smoking?
Who in your family smoked when you were a child?
Who in your family smokes now?
Is anyone in your family suffering from a serious
    chest condition?
Has anyone in your family died from a chest con-
    dition?
Do you know anyone who has died from or has a
    serious chest condition?
Do you smoke at a level that could kill you?
What is your most common feeling when you reach
    for a cigarette?
What might you be feeling if you didn't smoke?

How many times have you stopped smoking and
   restarted?
Do you intend quitting smoking?
When?
Have you a cough?
When?
Do you bring up any mucus?
Do you suffer with hay fever?
Do you suffer with sinusitis?
How many colds a year do you get?
Has that altered recently?

Have you any pain in the chest?
Do you exercise in a way that influences your
   breathing?

The Cardio-vascular System

Do your ankles swell?
Do you become short of breath without exercising?
Are you breathless when lying flat?
How much exercise do you do?
What is the nature of the exercises?
Have you any pain in the chest?
Do you suffer from palpitations?
At what times?
Have you varicose veins?
Have you ever had any heart problem?
Is your heart normal?
Has anybody in your family, when you were a child,
   suffered a heart attack or any other heart
   disease?
Did they survive?
Have you cold hands or cold feet?

The Musculo-skeletal System

Have you any aches or pains in any muscles, bones
 or joints?
If so, describe the areas affected.
How long have you had the pain?
Is it worse in the hot or cold weather?
Is the pain affected by the time of day or the
 amount you have exercised?
Have you had any X-rays taken?
Do you have them with you?
Is the pain affected by your diet?
Is there a family history of arthritis?
Have you any arthritis now or in the past?
Have you broken any bones?
To what do you attribute any musculo-skeletal pain?

The Genito-urinary System

How frequently do you pass urine in the day?
How frequently do you pass urine at night?
How much urine do you pass at these times?
Does passing urine cause pain?
Where is the pain?
What is the nature of the pain? (burning or
 scalding)
What is the color of your urine?
Does the color vary?
According to what?
Is there a slight tingling in the urethra when you
 urinate?
Is the urine cloudy?
Is the urine foul-smelling?

Have you any pain in your loins? (If so, the pain
   questions follow.)

Women

Have you ever suffered from cystitis?
When, and how often?
Do you have a vaginal discharge?
What is the nature of the discharge? (color, con-
   sistency, odor)
How long have you had it?
Do you have symptoms with the discharge?
Does intercourse affect those symptoms?
Have you had vaginal infections in the past?
When was your last smear test?
What was the result?
Do you suffer from herpes?
If yes, to what degree?
For how long?
Under what conditions?
With which partners?
What treatments have you tried?
What do you feel when you have an attack of
   herpes?
Are you having menstrual periods?
Are they regular?
How frequently do you have them?
How long do they last?
Do you use tampons or external pads?
How many of these might you use during the first
   few days, and over the whole period?
Do you lose excessive quantities of blood? (menor-
   rhagia)
Do you have pain?
Describe the pain.

Finding the Cause

Is the pain excessive? (dysmenorrhea)
Is that pain a problem for you?
Is the pain made worse by intercourse?
If your periods have finished, how old were you at
  the time? (menopause)
How old were you when you had your first period?
  (menarche)
Have there been times when your periods were light
  (oligo-menorrhea) or absent? (amenorrhea)

Have you any children?
What were the births like?
Have you ever miscarried?

(A more detailed obstetric history is taken in the
event of an obstetric problem, for example, failure to
conceive.)

Are you currently having intercourse?
How often do you have intercourse?
How many sexual partners do you have?
Do you have orgasms with intercourse?
Do you masturbate?
How often?
Do you have orgasms from masturbation?
Are your sexual partners men, women or both?
Which do you prefer?
Do you like men's genitals?
Do you like women's genitals?
Describe what you like about them.
Describe what you don't like about them.
Describe your own genitals.
Are you married?

Do you practice any contraception?

What sort and for how long have you used that
method?
Are you aware of the time you ovulate?
Do you menstruate or ovulate on the full moon?
Do you menstruate at the same time as other
women in your household?
Is your current method of contraception satis-
factory?

Men

Have you any discharge from your penis?
If so, describe the nature of the discharge.
How long have you had it?

Do you suffer from herpes?
(If yes, the same questions as for women)

Is there any problem with your testicles?
When you pass urine, is there any dribbling once
you have stopped?
Do you feel like passing urine again soon after you
have urinated?
Is your urinary stream as good as it used to be?
Do you have any trouble initiating urination?
Can you urinate in front of other men with no
problem?

Are you currently having intercourse?
How frequently do you have intercourse?
Is your erection satisfactory?
Do you ejaculate satisfactorily?
Do you masturbate?
How frequently do you masturbate?
Do you have sex with men, women or both?

Finding the Cause

Which do you prefer?
Is your anus a sexual area for you?
Describe what you like about men's and women's
    genitals.
Describe what you don't like about them.
Describe your own genitals.
How old were you when you started/stopped having
    intercourse?
Are you married?

The Central Nervous System

Do you have headaches?
Describe them.
Where are they located?
How often do you get them?
When do you get them?
How severe are they?
What brings them on?
What eases them?
What medication do you take?
What role does your emotional state play in the de-
    velopment of your headaches?
What events in your life regularly precede them?
Who in your family as a child had headaches?
Who in your family now has headaches?
When did either of your parents tend to get their
    headaches?
What can you remember hearing about headaches?
Have you ever had them investigated? (X-rays,
    scans, blood tests, etc.)
Do your headaches incapacitate you for everything
    or some things only?
Why do you think you get headaches?
How can you get rid of them?

Do you sleep well or poorly?
If poorly, what's the problem?
Do you find yourself having difficulty getting off to
    sleep?
Do you wake up earlier than you would like?
Do you wake refreshed?
Do you usually sleep alone, or with someone?
At what time do you go to bed?
At what time do you rise?

Are you suffering from any disease of the central
    nervous system?
Do you have any unusual symptoms that you have
    been unable to explain?

Is your vision satisfactory?
Do you wear glasses?
When did you first need glasses?
How old were you at the time?
What was happening in your immediate family at
    that time? Was that a problem for you?
Has your eyesight been improving/deteriorating?

Is your sense of taste normal?
Is your hearing normal? (if no, same questions as
    for visual defect.)
Do you suffer from "pins and needles?"
Where?

Medication

List everything you are currently taking that is not
    a foodstuff.
(Include drugs prescribed by a medical practitioner,
herbal medicines, homeopathic remedies, miner-

als and tissue salts, vitamins, flower remedies,
naturopathic remedies, self-made medicines.)
How often and in what doses have you been taking
them?
How long have you been taking them?
How do they help you?

Social History

Do you live alone?
With whom do you live?
What is your relationship with the people you live
with?
Are they lovers, friends, acquaintances?
Are you in a relationship at the moment?
Are you happy in your current household?

What is the nature of your work?
Are you employed in the workforce as a salary
earner?
Are you self-employed?
How long have you been unemployed?
Is that through choice or unavailability of work?
What skills do you have?
What qualifications do you have?
Do you like your job?
Do you like being unemployed?

What is happening in your life at the moment?
What happened in your life a year ago?
Is there anything or anyone that you are missing?
Are you feeling generally happy, sad, angry or
afraid?

What thoughts regularly occur to you?

What relationship do your thoughts and feelings
  have to your illness?

Are you financially secure?

Do you consider yourself a spiritual person?
Do you belong to a religion?
Do you meditate?
What are your hobbies?
Have you enough friends?
Are you lonely?
What has happened in your family as a conse-
  quence of your illness?
What has happened to you as a consequence of your
  illness? (This inquiry is expanded in Chapter
  21—At Your Invitation Only, page 349.)

The Diet History

(I now go through the client's diet, asking first
what he eats, then what he drinks, asking for a
range of things, since each day may be different.)

What do you have for breakfast?
What time is that?
How long do you take to eat it?
What do you have for lunch?
What time is that?
How long do you take to eat it?
What do you have for a coffee break?
What time is that?
How long do you take to eat it?
What and when do you take snacks?
What do you drink? How much?

(The diet of one of my clients follows. I make no

comment on its suitability, but use it to demonstrate the detail necessary.)

8:00 a.m.—Breakfast

Muesli, homemade, with nuts, almonds, cashews, sunflower seeds, raisins, oats, millet, rye, wheat.
Milk on the muesli.
Honey from the supermarket on the muesli.
Toast, whole-wheat. Butter, unsalted. The bread is from the local health shop. Peanut butter or marmalade.

10:30 a.m.

Apple or banana.

1:00 p.m.—Lunch

Whole-wheat bread roll with cheese, lettuce and beet, or whole-wheat sandwich with coleslaw, carrot, cabbage and tahini.
One whole-wheat cracker.
An apple, or in season grapes, apricots or peaches.

4:00 p.m.

A cracker with either cheese, tomato or both.

7:00 p.m. — Evening meal

Who prepares it?
Meat—steak three times a week, chicken three times a week, lamb occasionally, fish once a week.

Brown rice—once every two weeks.

Legumes (soy beans, lentils etc.) occasionally.

Vegetables, cooked (boiled usually, sometimes in
  safflower oil, Chinese style) potato, pumpkin,
  beans, peas, cabbage, carrot, ginger, garlic.
  Vegetables, raw—lettuce, tomato, carrot, cabbage,
  parsley, cucumber, radish, capsicum, celery,
  green beans, mushroom, endive, bean sprouts,
  garlic.

Desserts—the occasional apple crisp with ice cream,
  fresh fruit in season.

Drinks—in cups per day:
  Tea (ordinary) milk, no sugar—two
  Coffee (milk, one sugar)—four
  Tea (herbal), rosemary, peppermint,
  chamomile—one
  Coffee substitutes—occasionally
  Fruit juice—-three
  Cordial—none
  Mineral water—occasionally
  Tap water—two
  Alcohol—one glass white wine most nights, on
  weekends six glasses of beer and maybe some
  spirits. Two bourbons and three gins on both
  Friday and Saturday.

Dairy products— rated between + and + + + according to the tone of the voice. For example,
  "Do you drink much milk?" may be answered
  by, "Oh, a little." The inflection on the "oh" will
  give an idea of the amount consumed. The reply
  to "How much butter do you eat?" could be
  "Oh, not much." This "oh" will sound quite
  different.
  Milk + +
  Cheese + +

Yogurt + +
Cream + +
Butter + +
Chocolate
Ice cream + + +
Fruit—fresh per day three to four pieces
Dried + +

Nuts + +
Salt +
Pepper +
Curries, spices + + +
Herbs + +
Honey + +
Sugar +
Eggs per week—three
Sweets—two muesli bars from the health shop each
    week.

Is there anything else that you regularly eat that I
    haven't covered here?

Those are all the questions I have at that point, although I tell the client to feel free to ask any other
questions, or to mention anything that's not been covered. I now move on to the physical examination, asking the client to remove his clothing completely and
lie on his back on the couch, indicating a blanket if he
wishes to cover himself. I leave the room for a moment
while the client undresses. If he's consulted me before
and isn't bothered by undressing in front of me, I may
stay and continue the conversation. The client's reaction to taking off his clothes is obviously of importance
in establishing his body image, that it, how he feels
about his body and about other people seeing it.

The Physical Examination

I do the orthodox examination first, followed by the
    acupuncture, naturopathic and psychosomatically
    orientated examinations.
I record the following:
Blood pressure
Pulses
Heart rate
Auscultation of (listening to) the heart
General blood circulation
Varicose veins
Breathing pattern
Auscultation of the chest
Percussion (tapping),
    palpitation (feeling) of the chest
General shape of the chest wall
General oxygenation of the tissues
Mouth
Tongue color, and the distribution of a pattern, if
    there is one.
Odor Tonsils Fauces (cavity at the back of the
    mouth)
Palate
Gums
Teeth (I look very carefully at each tooth and note
    if there are fillings. I note the type of material
    the fillings are made from, and if they extend
    below the gum margin. I ask about any root
    canal therapy. I look for any uneven wear of the
    teeth, and note if the person is grinding away
    the tooth enamel or the filling, indicating anxi-
    ety or anger. I return to the desk and write

down the findings before proceeding.)

The lymphatic system I examine by feeling for glands in the neck, beneath the arms and in the groin area.

In women, I next palpate the breasts.

The abdomen is next palpated.

I feel for the major organs, liver, kidneys, spleen, bladder, womb.

I feel for the intestines, stomach and colon and take some notice of the epigastric area (looking for heartburn).

I examine the genitals in both men and women after I have indicated that I wish to do so.

Men

Penis, circumcised or not, state of foreskin, cleanliness of area, feeling the whole length of the urethra for pain and inflammation. Looking for old or new herpes scars. The shape and size of the penis. If I notice him getting an erection, which is quite common, especially in young boys, then I say something like, "You'll probably get an erection during this examination, that's normal, don't bother about it." If he does sustain an erection, I note the size of his erect penis. The testicles are palpated and examined.

Women

I am more hesitant about the examination of women because of the risk of prosecution by someone intending to harm me. This is unfortunate but I make no apology for looking after myself first. In practice, I can usually tell if there will be a problem and in those circumstances, omit part of the examination. Otherwise, I examine the external genitalia, labia, clitoris, vaginal opening, urethral opening. I note if there is mucus secretion, its nature, and whether it's a consequence of sexual excitement. If I need a specific examination of the internal organs, I will perform a vaginal examination with the woman's permission.

If there has been an indication, either a symptom or a sexual practice, which the client has mentioned, I will examine the anus. Other orthodox examinations, such as rectal examinations, are performed when indicated or for prophylaxis (prevention).

The eyes, ears, and nose are all examined when indicated, and on all occasions in children. Similarly, the central nervous system will be examined when there is a problem in that area.

I will next ask the client to stand up and face the wall away from me. I look at the general dimensions of the body, the amount of fat, the spine, the broadness and straightness of the shoulders. I look at the size and shape of the legs and buttocks and the general body posture. I then ask him to turn side on. The protuberance of the abdomen, chest, breasts, buttocks and spine are best viewed from here. I then stand about six meters from him and examine him from the front. The general way clients feel about themselves is best seen from this angle. Stooped shoulders, one shoulder higher than the other, thrusting forward of the breasts or genitals, holding in of the waist, etcetera, are all noted. Next the client returns to the face-down position on the couch and I examine the back, looking for spinal adjustments that may be possible or desirable in the future and feeling the musculature available to me in that position. When I touch the buttocks I note the degree to which clients attempt to protect their anus by clenching their buttocks. The amount of muscular tension (or "armoring") is noted. This can also be seen in the muscles about the neck, shoulders and chest.

I may return the client to the face-up position to check something noted elsewhere, such as the tension in the chest muscles. I am looking for how much of this is chronic, and how much acute, and what appears available for change. I may look at the muscle tension on the inside of the thigh, which particularly in women, indicates sexual inhibitions. In men, external rotation of the feet indicates buttock contraction and sometimes fear of homosexuality. If some functional disturbance of the body musculature appears, the client is asked to adopt various positions so that this may be more fully assessed. For example, the client may bend backwards to assess the flexibility of the spine. Very often he's asked to walk up and down the office.

If I suspect that the client is really very sad and struggling to conceal it, then I may press quite hard on the area that looks to be carrying the load of that suppressed emotion. This is very often the chest muscles in both men and women, and firm massage of that area will usually result in the person bursting into tears. If I do that, I need time to handle the situation, so naturally I pick my time. Generally, body work will not be done during this first session.

By now, I have a pretty complete impression of the overall body shape of the person, and can move onto more specific areas. Just as the face represents the underlying personality exactly, so I believe does the body.

Next I take notice of various proportions, for example, the head compared with the shoulders, the ears compared with the eyes, the relative size of the left and right breast, the upper limb musculature compared with the lower limbs. The right and left side of the body are of considerable interest to me—which side is hypertrophied, which side is thrust forward, which side is the more active or the more irritable? At the same time that I'm paying attention to this I'm hearing in his speech and noting from his sphere of interests whether he's a right- or left-sided person. Functionally, it may be evident by one side of the face being more flexible than the other. Much has been made in acupuncture for thousands of years about left- or right-sidedness and for a hundred or so years in homeopathy, but only relatively recently has Western psychology given the notion much credence. It is of importance in choosing the medium for communication and subsequent treatment of any individual. We are dealing here, in the broadest terms, with the symmetry of an individual's personality.

The degree to which the mind has instructed the body in its development of the years is the next area of interest. I pay particular attention to the nutrition of the various parts, believing that if the skin is shining, the muscles are powerful and flexible, the tendons are supple, and all parts enjoy a good blood supply, then the mind has an investment in those areas being strong. If the blood supply is poor, the skin dry and lifeless, the contour indecisive and the tone limp, I assume that the mind has not put much energy into developing that area and that the individual feels safer with the part undeveloped. Such an imbalance of one area of the body guarantees an imbalance elsewhere. It's not a difficult task, using the techniques of yoga, autogenic training or meditation, to increase the blood supply to particular areas of the body. The feet I have found to be very reliable in providing a general impression of whether the person wants to be upright and mobile. Beautiful, well-nourished feet are to me both delicate and powerful sculptures.

The client's reaction to this examination is monitored continually. Reluctance to undergo some parts of the examination, as with reluctance towards some of the inquiry, is clearly significant. I may choose to investigate this reluctance by pressing on, or backing off and coming back later. In general terms, a balance is struck between taking the client's fears into account (and these are usually obvious) and confronting them. That requires an intuitive feel for the client's awareness. If the practitioner oversteps the mark then she can expect to lose that client. Interestingly, middle-aged women who have never masturbated or discussed their sexual activity with anyone, and whom I thought would have found the topic indelicate, usually welcome a full discussion of the art of clitoral stimulation and an anatomy lesson of the area.

That's the end of the physical examination for the first session, and the client is asked to get dressed. If some emotional catharsis has occurred and the client is indicating he would like a hug, then I may hug him. This is unusual so early in our relationship but people come to therapy in various stages of preparedness.

The information I've gathered is on two levels. First, I have written down the result of the orthodox examination on the case notes and some of the other information as well. The majority of it is stored in my conscious and subconscious where it will be recalled and reprocessed when I see the client next and the story continues. Much of this information I will not even be aware of in the first session.

Occasionally I will have time to recommend dietary prescriptions on this first visit, but often this must wait until we meet again. By this time the client will generally feel safer with me. We agree to reconvene the meeting. This next meeting will either be for an hour or a half-hour. During that time I will collate and summarize my findings. I'll then make some recommendations at the level we've reached so far. The next stage will be the offer of further inquiry into the underlying causes of the disease. This involves both establishing the advantages of the immediate illness and the psychological inquiry, or so-called "Script Questionnaire."

The first interview with the client has taken one hour. From the amount of data that I've been describing, it's clear that the pace of the interview is considerable. I would really like to take two hours for this initial contact, but the expense becomes prohibitive to a client relying on an often hostile insurance company for reimbursement. There's no need to go into all the areas that I've mentioned with every client on the first visit. Indeed, with some of them, they never get investigated. Alternatively, the examinations mentioned represent a broad overview. For specific clients and specific conditions, more specific inquiry and examination is warranted. I may become sidetracked very early on in the interview and spend the whole hour dealing with the client's immediate domestic situation. Generally, I adopt the attitude that if the client, who is as aware of the restrictions of time as I am, chooses to remain on the one topic, she may do so. If I think she's using one topic of conversation to avoid more important and more sensitive areas, I'll confront her with that. Usually the energy of the client will be centered on her problem, so I'll go with her.

8

Family Needs
Become Physical Diseases

GENERALIZED CONCLUSIONS FROM
THE EXAMINATION DATA

The comments that follow are my own. I have come to believe them by observing myself and a group of people for whom they are true, or were true. In that sense they are both subjective (from observing myself) and empirical (from observing others). In the future they cannot be relevant in exactly their current form because times and people change. So too will my interpretation of the data.

Personal Details

Title

I don't ask women for a title directly. If they offer one, then I write it down. I'm not interested at this point in their marital status, in fact often it's not relevant at any point. If they are married and use the title Ms., then they have defied convention and that may represent an effort, rebellion, or a new attitude to themselves or their husbands. Men always call themselves Mr. and that's not much help in telling me what they think of themselves. I take note of the title medical practitioners use.

Name

The name is always of great significance, although since I have no way of getting inside the head of the parent who chose it, I may not be able to use it fully. Eric Berne, in his book *What Do You Say After You Say Hello?*, Grove Press, New York, 1972, details the significance of names. Here are some simple examples. If a boy is called Robin or Pat, or if a girl is called Jo or Ronnie, then I look for gender identification, that is, in what proportions has the person adopted masculine and feminine traits?

Usually such clients will display characteristics of the opposite sex more obviously than people with unambiguous names like John or Rosemary. If you doubt this, think of the people you know and match their personalities with their names or, more accurately, the names they go by. The feminine characteristics men display may vary between the extremes of female impersonation on the one hand and sewing on the other, and are feminine or not according to one's own frame of reference. The ambivalence of the parent or parents towards having a boy or girl is embodied in the sexually ambivalent name. As such it's usually of little consequence (heaven help us if we were all Johns or Rosemarys) but it alerts me to the client's willingness to be open to both men and women.

Women called Peta who were the third born in an all-girl family and whose father longed for a boy, may find themselves raised as a son, and unwilling to be vulnerable with men. They may have light menstrual periods, that often cause imbalance in the genito-urinary system, and fatigue. In such cases, I question whether they have accepted being a female and if their hormonal levels have been affected by that decision. I make the point that names are of some significance.

Age

Needless to say the age of the client is of paramount importance in any sensible diagnosis and treatment. It is absolute nonsense to treat a fifty-year-old as you would treat a fifteen-year-old. The aging process is relentless and cannot be stopped. Nevertheless, the orthodox profession pays little attention to age and may be found treating a five-year-old with tonsillitis in exactly the way they treat a sixty-year-old. To my mind that's ridiculous. The treatment will depend to a large degree on the age of the client. Teenagers who have not finished rebelling against parents are different from twenty-year-olds who have, and from five-year-olds who haven't started yet and are totally dependent on parents.

From a knowledge of age, the aging process may be assessed. Someone who enjoys being alive and celebrates his body will be less affected by age and be less ill than a person who is unsure he was ever meant to be alive and has yet to decide he'll live. The decision to retain death as a prominent option, or an ambivalence towards life, is often a major consideration of therapy. Why bother to decide to be well if you haven't yet decided to live?

Address

The address will sometimes inform me of the financial state of the client, or of his appreciation of trees, the seaside, the mountains or the countryside. If he informs me later that he doesn't like living where he is or he's about to move, then I ask why. Children can usually tell you their address by the time they are four or five.

Number of Children

People who have raised their own children or have been in close contact with others who have children have a different perspective on some things. The difficulties involved in raising our own children often help us to appreciate the even more harrowing circumstances under which we were raised. We get a new perspective on all the "wrongs" we feel from childhood and this often proves invaluable when the time comes to forgive our own parents for the racket feelings we have held onto. As previously mentioned, the racket feelings are those feelings not coming from immediate circumstances but from incidents in the past. They eat away at the mind and the body, are seen clearly in the face and physique of the person, and must be dropped if a cure of the disease is intended.

Parents may be either more or less receptive than people without children to the notion that children adapt very quickly to parental demands. Children may comply or rebel. Often when they appear to be compliant, they may secretly be rebellious. Parents understand these things, seeing them every day. It often takes a lot more talking to convince a non-parent that children are responsive to the most subtle changes in the family and that illness is one of the ways they learn to manipulate their environment. Young children have no direct control over their lives because they cannot keep themselves alive independently, and in this situation are much more aware of other ways to get what they want. Being sick is a favorite, condoned as it often is by the parents themselves.

On the other hand, some parents will not admit the game their children are playing around illness, as it would be very frightening for them to admit either the same game themselves or their conspiring role that keeps it going, that is, encouraging the children to be ill so that the parent can fulfill a caring role. They may still be playing "I'm not in control of my life," and this may interfere with their acknowledgement of how they make themselves ill. Either reaction, the acceptance through personal fear of the role of early childhood conditioning, is significant. Hence, I like to know if clients have children of their own.

The Presenting Complaints

By the time clients have talked about their condition in some detail, either volunteering information or answering questions, their general attitude to illness will be recognizable. It is once again both what they say and how they say it. They aren't led when describing the presenting complaints. If they leave out relevant information, then clearly they don't consider it to be relevant (or don't want it to be) and this is often a clue where to look next. For example:

> "Doctor, my eyesight has been failing me recently."
> "How long has it been a problem, Mrs. White?"
> "I'm not sure, Doctor, a few months maybe."
> "What happened to you a few months ago, anything significant?"

Finding the Cause

After a few moments, in which the client attempts to conceal the fact that she's crying, she tells me her husband died six months ago and she's finding the grieving difficult.

Now this demonstrates a few things. Give clients time and permission and in their own way they will assess whether the doctor is receptive to the real story, and if so, will tell him. Secondly, the presenting complaint is very often a minor complaint, mentioned first for safety. If the doctor is frightened by the emotional aspects of an illness, clients will often take care of the doctor by not mentioning it. In reality this is taking care of themselves by reaffirming their view of the medical profession as unsympathetic, that is, "nobody can help me." My advice to clients is that if they have something they want to tell a helping professional then tell him. Any discomfort on the part of the professional is for him to deal with.

Those people who believe that their problem is the result of bungling on the part of the medical profession or others will usually have considerable energy available with which to discuss (condemn) previous doctors, diagnoses and treatments. They're less keen to discuss the role that they've played in their illness. Some of course have a valid case against incompetent doctors, particularly when they were children and unable to pick a doctor for themselves.

I assess adults' needs to choose medical practitioners who are dangerous. We all have considerable intuition, and if we repeatedly consult a person on any matter and that person proves unworthy, then we aren't looking after ourselves. What do we say about ourselves when yet another medical practitioner proves to be useless, and how is being able to reaffirm that view an advantage? By such inquiry, awareness of the client's role in choosing an incompetent practitioner is established, and in most cases, anger towards the profession overlies anger towards one or both parents. This needs to be dealt with. Forgiveness of both self and parents, or "dropping the past," cures more illness than antibiotics ever will.

We have spoken before about the tone of voice, and how it may be profitably employed in establishing the psychological profile. It is nowhere more beneficial than here, when the client is describing an illness that is obviously of much distress to him. If he's in the habit of using his illness to manipulate others, the voice will often be powerless and pleading, wavering usually with the strains of life. Or it may be defiant, as in, "Yeah, well I'll bet you can't cure me!" And of course that's entirely accurate. Nobody can cure anybody else, especially if that person has declared himself incurable. It's the attitude to his illness that's initially important, not which particular physiological disturbance (disease) he has chosen with which to inconvenience himself. The attitude is evident through observation of all the body language, tone of voice, mode of expression. When his attitude to his illness is established, a program can be used to establish the needs being met by the illness and safer ways worked out to satisfy those needs. The particular illness decided upon by the client will suit his purposes exactly and at a later time will provide much insight into the individual's specific needs.

Medications

Current medications will give much information about the degree of self-responsibility the client considers reasonable. If she's taking a large quantity of orthodox prescription drugs, that's tantamount to putting her faith in the orthodox medical profession. (In the Western world the *average* person takes a medication most days of his or her life—see D. N. Darby, S. Glasser and I. F. Wilkinson in *Health Care and Lifestyle*, New South Wales University Press, Sydney, 1981. Staggering, isn't it?) By so doing, she has absolved herself from most or all of her responsibility to be her own guardian. In this she is heavily encouraged by her advisers, who react with fear if she does something not under their immediate control, especially when they know nothing about it. Some people who have no demonstrable pathology have been given over thirty medications a day, comprising some ten different drugs, by doctors too scared to inquire about the client's psychological state. I deal with such cases frequently. On a more common level, the number of people who survive on uppers and downers of all descriptions is frightening. Usually they are middle-aged rather than young, and their frustration with not being made happy by taking the medications is made obvious by the vitriolic attacks they direct at those who overtly take drugs and enjoy the experience.

Or the client may religiously avoid prescription drugs but take vitamin pills in large doses. Encouraged by those who dislike the orthodox profession and by the retailers of such pills, she believes that by taking doses of vitamins she's taking care of herself. She is not, at least in my experience. While I accept that for brief periods of time some people benefit from vitamins, the general trend to take high doses of all kinds is both useless and expensive. I regard much vitamin self-administration as no more than an individual clutching at straws intended to absolve him from being his own highest authority and, by keeping himself under the protective umbrella of the vitamin-pill manufacturer, guarantee the continuation of his dependence and his disease. Often these people are incredibly righteous. They don't take "nasty drugs," prescribed by the medical profession, they take homeopathic pills prescribed by their naturopath. Commonly they declare, "They can't do you harm, they can only do you good."

What rot! Anyone with the most elementary grasp of dialectics or paradox will tell you that if something is capable of healing it must also be capable of harming. Without such a grasp of Yin and Yang it becomes impossible to cure disease. Disease itself is one of the great paradoxes. It both helps and harms. Ignorance in these areas is widespread, and in this climate it becomes easy for the unscrupulous to prey on the fears of the public. "If you don't take a gram of vitamin C a day you're missing out on an essential ingredient of the diet!" is a common fallacy. The underlying message here is that by taking a gram of vitamin C a day, you'll be happy. I can report that the unhappiest group of people I see are the vitamin freaks. A little of what you want can't hurt you but to place a great deal of importance on taking large doses of vitamins is bound to disappoint.

Some people will be taking remedies handed down through the family, which they are often reluctant to mention for fear of ridicule. I encourage them to tell me about them, though, not only because this adds to my knowledge of the illness, but because I find the old remedies fascinating and use some of them myself. They are intervention to be sure but much more gentle. It's interesting to note the ways in which the old "flu" remedies vary from one country to the next, often only slightly if the countries are adjacent like Poland and Czechoslovakia. The remedies also vary between families. This is significant because illness begins within the family in the early days of the client's life, and old remedies usually reflect the parental attitude to illness. If this can be established, it's much easier to work out why the client wants to be ill. Warm honey and lemon, for example, may be conveying "I love you, dear, this'll make you feel better," while a mixture of ground root ginger, pepper, lemon peel and garlic would mean more "If you get ill then you have to take this vile mixture." The recipient of honey and lemon may be more inclined to repeat the experience than the latter.

Diseases that are really a consequence of the collective family mentality are often thought to be genetically inherited. Eventually they may become inherited but in the first place they are probably behavioral. That's why I gather as much information about the family as possible, and old remedies that the client still uses are both exciting and informative.

Herbal remedies are taken by people with such varying approaches to health that to conclude anything from the simple information that a client was taking them would be foolish. Further inquiry is required to establish whether they are being used as a panacea, which they certainly are not, or with the sophistication and the real value that results from them being used symptomatically with prudence. To take something every day of your life because someone has told you that you need it is nonsense. To occasionally take a herb in order to abate a troublesome symptom while looking for the root of the problem is valuable.

What Do You Think The Problem Is?

If the client doesn't volunteer this information then I request it. I'm interested if she pushes her view of the illness, or if she has an opinion that she's concealed from all the practitioners that she's attended, fearing their ridicule. It's not easy to maintain that your tinnitus is worse when your husband comes home drunk and violent, if the medical officer and the union representative are all pushing the line that it's an industrial injury and eligible for compensation.

I believe clients know the origins of their illnesses. Deep inside will remain a vestige of awareness of what role the illness played when it was chosen, what it did for them then and what it's doing for them now. In giving clients the opportunity to express their views, I can assess how much they have been prepared to examine their lives in trying to heal themselves, and therefore how afraid they are. Such an assessment will be relevant in deciding at what level and at what time to pitch the cure. Psychological training is unnecessary for a very sophisticated appraisal of the underlying psychodynamics, as the two following examples in which clients provide their own analyses demonstrate.

A man consulting me about his cancer started by telling me a family story surrounding his birth. This was unsolicited. The story was that his mother had tried to abort him by driving over rough roads. He figured he was an unwanted child, or at least ambivalence had surrounded his birth, and that was the reason for him deciding to give himself cancer and die. He reported that he had never felt the unconditional right to be alive. Eventually that belief transformed itself into a physical disease capable of fulfilling the belief. People materialize both what they believe and what they fear. Another man who had cancer of the scrotum was very sexually repressed by his mother, and even though he was too guilty to be openly angry with her, knew that the suppressed anger had converted itself into the cancer. He expressed this without prompting by whispering in exasperation, "Now I've caught this she ought to be happy!" Needless to say I heard that, mumbled as it was.

Other people refuse to admit any knowledge of what ails them.

> "What do you think the problem is, Mr. Petersen?"
> "That's what I've come here to find out, Doc!"

Most people who come to see me have made a few preliminary excursions into their own subconscious before the appointment and are ready to let me help them take a few more steps, but if they haven't, then I respect the attendant fear and don't confront them initially. However, if they maintain a position of non-awareness and non-responsibility for too long, then I terminate the arrangement, or they do. Relief is the accompanying feeling for both of us. They may criticize me openly around town, but as that serves to deter a lot of other people who aren't ready to heal themselves either, it ends well.

What's Been Happening In Your Life Recently?

What a question this turns out to be sometimes. Once again, clients are given ample time to mention this themselves but if they show no inclination to do so, I ask them. O. C. and S. Simonton and J. Creighton, in their excellent book *Getting Well Again*, published by Bantam Books, New York, in 1980, indicated that in the eighteen months preceding the onset of cancer, a significant life event often occurred. This event was traumatic in some way and initiated or promoted the cancer. The death of a loved one is a good example. My belief is that the basis of disease is in childhood and that precipitating events, such as those alluded to by the Simontons, are the immediate circumstances used in the service of the old decision taken in childhood. In other words, the precipitating event is just one of a long string of events that have confirmed the decision taken in childhood about what sort of place the world is. Hence, a man who decided as a child that death was always an option if he became too miserable or lonely, may, in the event of his wife leaving him, contract cancer and die. On an unconscious level, the man whose wife leaves him has chosen a wife whom he knows will do just that, and knows also that the event will precipitate a crisis for him. He knows that one way out of that crisis is death. When a life event merely confirms a view that we hold about ourselves, others or the world, we have usually set that event up so that it becomes inevitable. Not everybody kills themselves with cancer when their wife leaves. For some that is not an option.

The personal circumstances that the client takes the opportunity to mention will be those he sees as the most significant. It's impossible for the practitioner to be a mind-reader. He can see the basic emotions, the body language, the underlying psychological state, but the histories responsible for those conditions will be extremely varied. Now in a way the immediate situation of the client's personal life is not significant, that is to say, isn't causative. We will see later how it's helpful. However, the details are usually of great concern to clients, as they look for rights and wrongs, and the best way to recover from a painful situation. Often they will talk of relationships, but they could just as helpfully be talking about the collapse of the stock market and their ensuing fear and pain. The actual trauma is of importance only in that it provides a medium whereby the client's attitudes to life, himself, his relationships and his illness may be examined. The immediate situation will be remedied by remedying the underlying imbalance in his life, otherwise it, like illness, will recur.

In the case of personal relationships the situation may be beyond salvation and the parties must come to terms with losing someone they have cherished; then they need to grieve. Next time round they may choose someone different and consequently have no need for the migraine headaches that they chose to suffer from when their last lover came home late from work. In fact, if they feel safe enough after therapy they may choose not to suffer at all. Such is the range of available options. Illness and relationships are like motor cars: you choose the one you want. When one has served its purpose, you trade it in for another more suited to your current needs. Some people pick a suitable one first time.

In the most general terms, an individual who has a happy personal life, is financially secure and has achieved a level of spiritual grace is unlikely to be very ill, especially if she is about to take a holiday yachting about the Caribbean. On the other hand, someone who has come into a patch of "bad luck"—his business has gone bankrupt, his relationship is stormy and he's working too hard or not at all—is more likely to be seen looking and feeling ill. When a client tells me that everything in his life is wonderful and couldn't be better, and that the only thing bugging him is his recurrent bronchitis, I confess to not believing him. If he's convincing about being very happy, then I look at why he needs the pleasures of life to be interrupted by pain. Very often there will be a family background of achievement but an atmosphere of anxiety. The child becomes less afraid when the situation is anxious (Mom and Dad fighting usually), because that's what he's used to and he knows the rules. When things go right for him, he becomes scared. He may have no information on which to fall back in those good times and that is anxiety-provoking. In order to make himself feel safer he makes himself ill, not seriously, and not something that will interrupt his work too much, but some niggly little thing like an intermittent chest infection. Hence, the bronchitis. Awareness of the game will often be enough to change the behavior, although this may not happen immediately and may be punctuated by remissions or return to the old pattern. On the other hand, someone who tells me that everything in his life is perfect I may distrust, seeing the agony on his face, and ask about his need to be seen to be functioning perfectly when he is not.

Medical practitioners have incidents in their lives as well as clients, and these are often accompanied by a change in perspective by the doctor. The perception of the illness by the doctor will be different as her life unfolds. Needless to say, her treatments will also be constantly changing.

The Number And The Nature
Of The Presenting Complaints

Some people have ten complaints that they list in chronological order because they find them equally irritating. Others have one major complaint that they are not inclined to dilute with trivia. Others mention the worst complaint last, or hope that if they pay it little attention, it'll go away. Those who hope that I'll be put off and declare them to be incurable if they mention dozens of ailments will often fail to draw breath during their history for fear of an embarrasing question from me. By so doing, they hope to return home and declare to a spouse that the doctor was unable to help, whereupon they both breathe a sigh of relief. They employ a form of verbal barrage as their first line of defense. In Freudian terms, that's what illness is—an ego defense mechanism. What I'm observing is the life casualty, the stalwart or the fearful, and they're telling me, via a history of their illness, what their problem really is. I am listening.

The Past History

Some of this information is volunteered during the presenting complaint but much of it has little significance for the client, who therefore tends to omit facts that are essential in understanding how he's used illness in his life. The past history is a record of the early life decisions translated by the body into physical complaints. Usually the individual will have constructed life events that appear to correspond to the physical complaints, so that to the undiscerning the illness appears to have been triggered by external events beyond his control. Now some events to my mind are beyond our control, or very nearly. Famine, war, weather, epidemic diseases, other people's actions at times and earthquakes, to name a few, but most of the things that happen in our lives happen because we set them up. Often this is unconscious, reflecting a childhood decision about what we and the world are like. Having decided, for example, that the world was a dangerous place in which one was likely to be injured, an individual will put himself in situations in which that is made more likely and thereby fulfill that belief. He may loiter about places where aggressive individuals are known to congregate and where the odds of being assaulted are best. Or he may pick fights with people whom he suspects would react by giving him a beating. Why would anyone apart from a masochist get himself physically assaulted? He does it for excitement. This confirms he's alive. If a young boy is repeatedly hit by his father, and this constitutes the main interaction that the boy and his father have, in the mind of the boy, this is regarded as the essence of the relationship between himself and this man he loves. Since the boy is well aware in those early years that it's on the whim of his parents that he's provided for, the fear of being hit, staying alive and love become all the one thing, or confused. When as an adult the man gets himself physically assaulted, as he was in childhood, he is reaffirming his existence. In childhood, physical pain meant both love and existence as far as he was concerned.

It takes a lot to stop children from loving parents but when they do, it takes even more for them to forgive. For those who manage it, nothing is impossible. In essence, therapy revolves about the willingness to forgive. Before that happens, techniques that establish awareness of personal behaviors, and encourage expression of suppressed emotions, are employed.

What has all of this got to do with the past history of a medical inquiry? Those decisions that resulted in a man becoming a street-fighter rather than an astronomer, or a boxer rather than a beauty consultant, also determined that he suffers from heart disease instead of headaches, rheumatics rather than ruptures, and venereal diseases rather than ethereal diseases.

Finding the Cause

The frequency and severity of the diseases from which my client has suffered tell me whether the world has had its way with him, or he's had his way with the world. If he's been brought up with the clear instruction that he can take care of himself, then the latter will be the case. If he has no belief in his own power and is too frightened to use it, then he'll be suffering. He believes that the world is more powerful than he is and it can have its way with him. What he fails to realize is that the world can only have its way with him with his expressed permission. Usually he doesn't like to admit that permission has been given, however surreptitiously, and denies his power to even decide to be impotent.

Past Surgical History

> Appendix—age 9
> Tonsils—age 12
> Adenoids—age 15
> Submucous resection (for blocked nose)
>   —age 25
> Sinus washout—age 27
> Ovarian cyst—age 31
> Gallbladder—age 40
> Hysterectomy—age 45
> Varicose veins—age 47
> Vaginal repair—age 50

This is a typical surgical history in a fifty-year-old female who uses illness in her life as a way of manipulating her environment. It's a staggering price to pay for something she could have achieved more healthily had she and her advisers taken the time and effort to point out her role in those illnesses. If you think that the above list of operations is atypical, then ask a few women in that age-group and become enlightened about contemporary surgical practice. Each time an operation is performed there will be "very good medical reasons" for doing it. Any procedure can be justified if you choose a narrow enough frame of reference. Within the orthodox medical profession, despite magnificent achievements in both medical technology and surgical procedures, fear of the unknown is still very strong and keeps many doctors' frames of reference narrow. I believe their inflexibility stems from being regarded as omnipotent for so long; but today, the golden age of total faith in technology, or anything else for that matter, has gone. As I said previously, there's no guarantee that any operation performed these days is really necessary. I recommend that anybody who has been advised to have an operation gets a second opinion from someone with no investment in either the operation being performed or not being performed. Then listen to yourself.

In the case of the woman whose operations I have just listed, I suspect the notion that we create our own illness will meet with much anger. The anger will overlie the fear of change and of guilt at having used illness this way. It is essential (I will continue to repeat this) that the woman is congratulated on having worked out a way to get her needs met in as safe a way as possible for her. I don't condemn her for having multiple operations, in fact, quite the opposite. She's congratulated. There's also no condemnation of the surgeons for doing what they believed to be best. The majority of medical practice and the belief of the majority of the people about the nature of illness must be consistent. It's a mutual thing.

The fact that the woman with multiple operations has come to see me will often indicate that she's reached the conclusion herself that alternatives are required. If she's angry at her doctors for all the surgery, she'll be quite different from a woman who defends her advisers. In the first case she may be racket angry, still harboring old grudges against her parents; and in the second, she may be compliant, denying her anger and being sad instead.

A client may give a history of little surgery but a large number of medical conditions, over the years. Sometimes when a person is asked if she's had any operations, she becomes very indignant and righteously announces that "I have never had an operation in my life!" Meanwhile she may have a long history of swollen ankles, period pain, cystitis, backache, sinusitis, winter colds and sciatica to her credit. Obviously there's been some powerful parental injunction against having surgery but any number of medical complaints have been condoned. That, remember, is the child's interpretation of what she sees and hears from her parents about illness and wellness. It will also be reflective of the modeling that the child observes in her parents and others. If Mother has a headache when she doesn't want sexual intercourse, then the daughter may either comply with that use of illness and behave similarly, or reject that as an option and "never have headaches." In both cases the client is still in script, that is, still following those decisions taken as a child that were her best options then but could be bettered now that she can keep herself alive without her parents' help.

It's interesting to note whether the client accumulates treatments or if she moves onto the next condition when the old one is no longer useful. It has long been recognized in naturopathy that if a condition is suppressed, which is nearly always the case in orthodox symptomatic treatment, a new disease will eventually take its place. In my experience that is true. I think however that the changing needs of the client as well as her changing body physiology account for the giving up of one disease and the adopting of another. The suppression of acute diseases using drugs guarantees the later development of chronic diseases, as body physiology is interfered with in its attempt to complete an unfettered course of recovery. (See diagram on page 166.)

The role of illness in the life of any particular individual may not change dramatically, and yet we all know of people who have suffered many illnesses in their lifetime, some of which appear to be quite different from those that preceded them. I can think of some clients who are no sooner over one illness before they give themselves another. A person may decide to have asthma because he's afraid to live his life without his mother and his asthma attracts women to him who love looking after asthmatics (as did his mother). It may be that he needs some time off work and as a child the only time his father would allow him to stay away from school was when his asthma was severe. It may be that he has an important performance coming up at the auditorium and is scared of failing. He may be exceptionally angry with his wife for smoking inside the house and rather than tell her directly that he's angry, swallows the rage and gets asthma instead. He may be a teenage homosexual youth come to the city from a small country town, hoping to escape the persecution, and ending up with asthma every time he sees someone from his past. Or he may be a well-adjusted boy of nine with a family history of asthma so severe that he feels pressured into having it for a few years but has already made up his mind that in a short while he'll remove it forever. The same external

Finding the Cause

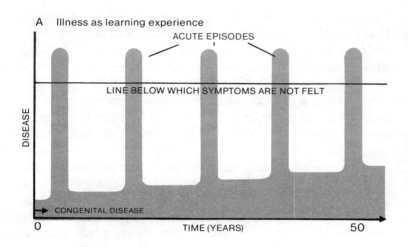

A Illness as learning experience

ACUTE EPISODES

LINE BELOW WHICH SYMPTOMS ARE NOT FELT

DISEASE

CONGENITAL DISEASE

0   TIME (YEARS)   50

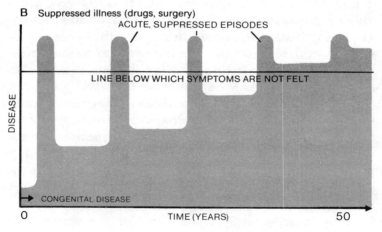

B Suppressed illness (drugs, surgery)

ACUTE, SUPPRESSED EPISODES

LINE BELOW WHICH SYMPTOMS ARE NOT FELT

DISEASE

CONGENITAL DISEASE

0   TIME (YEARS)   50

Where the body is supported in its efforts to heal itself (A), the level of disease returns to an acceptable level. At fifty years of age the amount of disease within the body, as represented by the shaded area on the graph, is small. Where drugs have been used to suppress the symptoms of acute episodes (B), the body never returns to its pre-existing state, but accumulates disease until symptoms are continually present. This is chronic disease. The shaded area in this case is far greater, making the cure of the illness much more difficult.

physical symptom, in this case asthma (constriction of the bronchial tubes), represents a myriad of underlying psychological profiles. The advantages in having asthma will be as numerous and as different as the individuals who suffer from it.

When a person's situation changes in any way, either by external factors beyond his control, such as a car accident in which a drunken driver caused a sudden and totally unavoidable collision, or by internal processes such as his reaction to the death of a parent, the need for the frequency, severity and the nature of illness may similarly change. Under such conditions, he may give up the usual illness, escalate it, trade it in for something more effective in the new circumstances, or give up the illness option altogether. And since we all grow older every day, our situation changes every day. The progression of illnesses that people who exercise the illness option choose to have is not surprising. A young man who needs hepatitis to keep him away from a sport he thinks he "should" play but which terrifies him, doesn't need to justify inactivity as he gets older. He may, however, need to justify a lack of promotion in his work. For this, chronic back pain is sufficient.

Childhood Diseases

This is a revealing section of the past history. In the most general terms those people who have been accustomed to illness as a child will continue to use it as an adult, that is, if you were sick as a child you'll probably be sick as an adult. Before the reader applies that generalization to his own case and finds it wanting, let me hasten to add that in human beings real change and maturity is no more spectacular than in the area of illness and wellness. Being ill or well is the mirror of the soul. Some people blossom from humble beginnings, others decay when they appear to have been given a head start. And so it is with disease. The sick child with a history of scarlet fever, polio, earache, encephalitis, glandular fever, mumps, chicken pox, rubella and epilepsy may reject all major diseases in adulthood and become an Olympic athlete. If he does this for himself, he can expect to remain well forever. If he's rebelling against his parents' use of illness (the system he adopted under pressure as a child) and still harbors a grudge, then he can expect to become ill again once the energy for being well to spite his parents has worn off and has been replaced by depression. In this case, he's not made a decision within a new frame of reference but has maintained the old belief system, that is, whatever happens to you as a child affects you for the rest of your life. Within the belief that nothing really changes, any number of options are available, none of which proves satisfactory. Sick children will become sick adults unless, from a position of self-love, they decide otherwise.

It has interested me that some nursing sisters appear to be very well when they're working and very sick when they retire. They have clearly been given the message in childhood to look after others, usually Mother herself, or a younger sibling, and in fear of not getting love may continue to follow the messages as adults and become nurses. If this is the case, that is, they are looking after others because they think it's the only way they are lovable, they will be afraid to become sick themselves. They are *supposed* to be taking care of patients. Although they are themselves well during their working life, their belief system is unchanged from childhood. They still believe as adults that to be loved requires selflessness and if you're unlucky enough to be ill, you get cared for. When they are old and haven't felt the closeness and caring that years of nursing were meant to provide, they become disillusioned, particularly if they have no family and are lonely. They are also angry at years of what they now regard as lost time. In this mood they become unwell, often seriously, and this means that someone has to care for them as they cared for others all those years. They frequently make terrible patients, demanding, aggressive, never satisfied and often alcoholic. Although they have been given "be well" messages, they have no permission to be well for others. When they become ill themselves, they do so within the same old framework.

I make the point that if illness is to be cured, some or all of the following need to happen: awareness ("So that's how I make myself ill!"), expression ("Damn you, Mom!"), forgiveness ("I accept the burden that raising six kids in the Depression must have been") and acceptance ("I love me, and I love others"). This means dropping the old belief system we adopted as children and taking full responsibility, without fear, for who we are.

Take the case of another nursing sister. Having found that this occupation that her mother had recommended was at times taxing, she decided that while at work she would care for the patients as their conditions warranted and get the caring she needed for herself at other times. She found herself a delightful lover, another nursing sister as it turned out, with whom she was mutually supportive. The two children of her lover's previous marriage were a source of joy to her. She allowed patients on the ward to do small things for her in return for the effort she put into their recovery. That effort was often directed towards showing them how they could reduce their dependance on their medical caretakers. This woman had no need to become ill, neither to confirm her right to caring nor to relate to her partner. She and her partner both believed in self-responsibility and mutual care within that responsibility. Both women in the first place had been encouraged to take up a caring occupation but both had subsequently decided that they could care and be cared for.

The frequency and severity of illness in childhood will reflect parental attitude to illness as well as genetic predispositions, birth trauma, environment and family diet, etcetera. If the individual continues to suffer multiple illnesses or at least continues with illness as an active part of his life, he's still adhering to the old decisions he made under external pressure as a child. If a man has been remarkably well following a sick childhood, then he may be rebelling against his parents, still hoping to get something from them that he didn't get as a child. "I'm going to be so damn well they'll realize their mistake and give me what I want." In this case he may end up sick, unhappy or both. Alternatively, he may decide that his earlier position no longer suits him and that in future he'll do things for his own sake. He can then expect to be generally well and occasionally suffer the minor irritations of a hostile environment until he's satisfied his will to live. When he's satisfied his will to live, presumably, he'll die.

The Family History

Having studied the prevalence of illness in the client as a child, we now turn our attention to the general family history. This reveals the parents' attitudes to their own state of health and provides more information on the sorts of messages the child would most likely have received. These can be compared with the client's recall of what they were directly told about illness, and where there are discrepancies, the reasons for them and their effect on the client can be assessed. This area is often of considerable importance in determining why people make themselves ill.

The ostensible or social message may vary substantially from the ulterior message. Take the following example: Joanne's mother was always ill. She was city-born and "just knew" she'd hate the country property where she and her country-born husband decided to live. Her daughter was born a few years later, and from the outset Mother had decided that this further imposition in life (the country was bad enough), was more than she could handle. She resolved to be unwell. This she did with a certain flair, for she had more than a touch of theatrics about her, and to the young Joanne such a display of infirmity had more than the desired effect. Her mother made it quite plain that Joanne was primarily responsible for her unhappiness; and for this, the girl would pay by attending her mother assiduously.

At the same time she was commanding attention and caring from Joanne, Mother would declare: "It's terrible being ill, dear, and the worst part is being a burden on you and your poor father. If there was one thing I could wish for you it would be good health, so that you wouldn't need others to take care of you." Any untoward thoughts that Joanne may have had about her mother's illness were easily engulfed by the wave of guilt she experienced at hearing her mother's words. How could she be so callous when the poor, sick woman only wished that she could stop being a burden on her family? What a trick to pull on a child or, more accurately, what an act of great hostility.

When Joanne came into therapy she was very angry at her mother, needless to say. She had developed herpes at the age of twenty and feared death from cancer of the womb. It had become almost an obsession. During the past history, I had elicited that as a child she'd been very well (in order to look after mother as it turned out), and without the family history, which she had omitted, a very incomplete picture of the case had emerged. The past history suggests messages about illness that would prohibit the child from being ill—"Don't be ill and be a burden on others"—but the modeling, or the ulterior psychological message from the mother, was quite clearly, "Life's a burden. You can ease it by getting ill and being looked after!" A combination of both the past and family history has made the situation very clear. The conflict had been, in Joanne, between the parent (grown-up) and the child (little kid) in her own head. While the parent said "Be well," the child sabotaged this with a "Be ill." She resolved this problem and developed into a beautiful woman once she learned to use her power to be well.

The family medical history is a record of the physiological responses of that family to the pressure of living. No doubt the reasons for the family as a whole being well or ill go back a long way, but for the purposes of investigating any particular client, the grandparents are as far into the past as we need go. Also, the general influence of the media is much stronger now than in the past and this is having a significant effect on attitudes to wellness, probably reducing the significance of the family. Still, television cannot keep babies alive.

During the family history I compare the state of health of the client with that of his siblings, his parents and his children. This further clarifies the overt and the ulterior messages. If I'm dealing with an obese client then I want to know who else in the family is overweight. Have his brothers and sisters similarly afflicted themselves, or was he singled out in some way? Was Mother obese from over-eating, under-exercise, sexual repression, a need for power or none of the above? As a child was he sickly, and did his mother become scared and overfeed him? In the latter case, the older siblings will probably be of normal weight, while the younger ones may have decided, like him, that it's dangerous to be thin.

Often I ask a sibling, a parent or a child to come and see me so that I can get a different perspective on the client's illness. In addition, this enables me to see and point out to the child the mechanisms that have resulted in illness in the parents, and therefore, if he's willing, steer him clear of the same dangers. That's preventive medicine. It's both exciting and sad to see how the client must have looked himself as a youth of nineteen. Eliciting the scripting is made so much easier by such experiences. In this case it's unlikely there's a genetic component to his obesity. Instead, he took a decision years ago that, "When I get older and lose the beauty of youth, I'll grow fat." There's a good chance the son will do the same thing.

Statements made in the family about people who were "always ill" or less often "always well" are of much value in determining the scripting and the racket feelings the client may have about his illness. If the client himself uses metaphors or cliches such as "Ah well, mustn't grumble," or recalls that a parent used them, his resignation towards life and illness is made so much clearer. I'm reminded in this of my grandmother, who would religiously inform me, "Your health is the most valuable thing you have, dear."

Listening to every metaphor, family saying, social platitude and frivolous comment, usually passed off with a laugh, is invaluable in eliciting the reality of that with which I'm dealing. Every nuance, every inflection of the voice is of great importance. It's the subconscious of your client telling you what he really believes, and what he'd like you to know, despite his protests to the contrary. Ask yourself if there are some stories or sayings that you recall from relatives about health, and if there are, look at them *literally*. They may help you to understand your own need for illness, as illustrated in the following example of the woman who remained happy and well as long as her husband remained alcoholic. When he dried out, she went to hospital with pleurisy. "Mom always said that if Dad came home from the pub sober just once, she'd die of fright!"

9

System Specificity: Which Disease Best Fulfills My Needs?

GASTRO-INTESTINAL SYSTEM

Both women, and to a lesser degree men, in Western society, have been brainwashed in the area of weight and sexuality. There are very few women of any age who do not regard the process of weighing as either a moment of great trial or of great triumph. For obese people, it's the moment of both shame and relief. They are ashamed of their "weakness," subconsciously needing to affirm that they're not OK, and simultaneously relieved to find that they still have their "complaint." People are the exact weight they want to be.

When people consult me complaining of obesity, I won't see them unless they agree to psychotherapy, in conjunction with diet, lifestyle, exercise, and meditation counseling. People choose a weight that is safe for them. Why should being a "perfect" weight be unsafe for anyone? This is a reasonable question, given the social acclaim that accompanies such a state. The following case demonstrates why it wasn't safe for one woman to be of normal weight.

Finding the Cause

When Jessica was two days old she had a seizure. Thirty-five years ago county hospitals were less sophisticated than they are today, and in the frustration of not knowing what caused it, and then what to do about it, the matron of the hospital informed Jessica's mother that the child had nearly died through lack of sufficient nourishment. (Babies hardly eat anything in the first two days of life anyway.) The accuracy of the information was less relevant, as was the ill-considered timing, than Jessica's mother's own internal needs to have a fragile child. What made her mother take such a drastic option I don't know, but she took it, with the result that young Jessica was overfed and grossly overweight from an early age.

At the slightest hint of an ailment, however minor, Mom would overfeed Jessica. In turn the child had few options in the situation. She could refuse to over-eat and perhaps withstand the threat from her mother to "eat or be ill," if her mother had little investment in the situation and was merely repeating what her mother had told her. But that wasn't the case. Young Jessica didn't have the maturity to handle the tension in the household if her mother was afraid. And her mother was terrified if Jessica didn't eat, believing that some disaster was imminent. As a consequence of Jessica taking care of Mother's fears and subsequently over-eating, she was quite gross by the age of twenty. I saw her when she was thirty-five. She came into my office accompanied by an older woman with whom I had no contact but guessed was her mother. Her mother's weight was normal, and after a short conversation with her daughter, it was mutually decided that Mother would remain in the waiting room and not accompany Jessica during the interview. By this stage, before a word had been spoken, the astute observer had diagnosed gross obesity (no prizes for that), with a considerable maternal investment. Now there aren't too many cases of obesity without a large maternal investment, but you don't often get to see it played out before you. Asking how Mom and Dad individually feel about having a fat daughter will indicate which of the parents is most significant in the client's decision to be overweight.

So great were her mother's fears that when Jessica married in her early twenties and moved to England to live, her mother followed and moved in with her daughter and son-in-law and proceeded to do all the cooking—in excessive quantities of course. Eventually the husband, who clearly liked grossly obese women but not, apparently, their mothers, could no longer stand the intrusion and moved out. Jessica and her mother moved back to Australia, took an apartment together, and once again the old routine of Mother overfeeding her daughter began. Of course, all of this happened with the approval of Jessica, who wasn't prepared to confront her own fears, made more acute no doubt by the presence of her real mother. If her mother hadn't been there, the situation would probably have been little different. Jessica would simply have maintained the fear of dying if she didn't eat from her own internal parent and child ego states. Her parent would say, "You should eat or you'll get sick!" while the child would regard the situation from a survival point of view. Hence, the power of the early childhood messages to continue dictating behavior as an adult.

Jessica had clearly decided that she couldn't stay alive without being overfed by her mother. She still believed that unless she was obese, she would die. She'd been told that the way to stay well was to be fat, and therefore believed that if she lost weight she was risking becoming ill. This is an example of keeping unwell in order to stay well. Such paradoxes need to be understood if a cure is to be attempted. The alternative (and this will be familiar to many readers), is to spend a fortune and often a lifetime on the merry-go-round of dieting and weight loss, frustration, over-eating, more weight gain and more dieting. After awhile the dieting makes little or no difference to body weight anyhow. The physiology of this has been discussed in The Childhood Basis of Disease on page 44.

Therapy centered on Jessica breaking her early childhood decision to be fat in order to help Mother feel comfortable, and taking responsibility for keeping herself alive. The decision to be both healthy *and* of normal weight was augmented by a program of healthy living and eating. We will be looking at treatment programs more specifically in a later section.

This case is a good example of psychological medicine working in an area that is very poorly catered for by the orthodox methods used in general practice. Very few cases of obesity are referred to psychiatrists or psychotherapists for treatment. The majority are given a diet, that doesn't work in the long term, or worse still, an appetite suppressant. Little more than such poor treatment is possible in the time spent with the average general practitioner. This is a pity because the average general practitioner is in the job because of both her interest and skills in the area of family and psychological medicine.

THE BOWELS

Within the systems inquiry, two specific areas are available for scrutiny of the internal functions, the bowels and the kidneys. In these areas we are able to assess the internal processes by observing and testing the excreta. By matching our findings with the psychological state, a direct method for assessing the body-mind axis is available. This is invaluable, so I spend much time inquiring about the exact nature of these functions. Most people find ten questions about the nature of their feces amusing, some are offended by the inquiry. Of course, their reaction is informative, as the following conversation shows:

> "How many times a day do you use your bowels, Peter?"
>
> "Normal."
>
> "Well, for you, how many times each day is that, on average?"
>
> "Oh, you know, normal!" He is becoming agitated. I press on.
>
> "Some people go to the toilet once a week, and for them that's normal, others go three times a day. I'm wondering where you fit into that range?" By this time I'm pretty sure that the answer will be "Once a week." "Well, if it's important, I suppose I go about once every few days, yes, about two or three times a week." Well, I was wrong about the frequency, but the quite severe constipation of his bowel reflects his mental constipation, not to put too delicate a point on it.

The bowel is an eight-meter-long, hollow, smooth, muscular tube. It's very susceptible to emotional changes, as anybody suffering from a stomach ulcer, heartburn, or irritable bowel syndrome (spastic colon) will tell you. It's classically affected in people who conceal their emotions, particularly anger and fear. The fact that they are reluctant to express their emotions may already be evident in other areas such as voice, dress, body shape, physiognomy, use of language.

The client's attitude to being questioned about his bowel function is an important indicator of the emotional climate that surrounded his early toilet training. Freud says the "anal stage" overlaps the "oral stage" (between birth and about eighteen months) and lasts until about three years. Children are usually toilet trained in this period, often quite aggressively, and issues stemming from that sort of treatment may result in individuals who are narrow in outlook, punctual in attendance and fastidious. They are usually suffering from lower-bowel problems, especially those closer to the anus such as irritable-bowel syndrome, hemorrhoids or cancer of the rectum. They aren't going to recover from those diseases until they're prepared to free themselves up and adopt a more *laissez-faire* attitude to life. This is often really scary for them, but it's my experience that if they take the plunge, they are very rewarding clients indeed. The change in their face is beautiful to see, more relaxed, more open, more accepting. If I need more information, I may insert my finger into the anus during the physical examination. If the anus is tight and very unwilling to be penetrated, then the same can be assumed of the psyche, impenetrable, with much protection or "ego defense."

The nature of the feces informs me of the diameter of the anus during defecation, and hence the degree of spasm. The consistency is indicative of the diet and the degree of digestion: a person who does not want to be nourished for fear of surviving may have intestinal hurry, loose, frequent bowel motions with undigested material visible. If the bowel motion floats in the toilet, then its specific gravity is lower than that of water and the fat content will be higher than normal, indicating that for some reason the liver is not removing the usual amount of fat from the food ingested. This often indicates a state of suppressed anger, a condition that I have found, and that is confirmed by acupuncture, as causing dysfunction of the liver. Hence the nature of the excrement may tell me why the client has arthritis (here a consequence of suppressed anger), a condition with apparently no connection to the bowel at all.

The bowel is the main organ with which we directly relate to our environment. The skin and the sense organs also relate to the outside world but in a more passive way. If we do not wish to see or hear something then we can interfere with the reception of these organs by decreasing their sensitivity. This way we become more dependent on our own internal processes, the external stimuli having been reduced. If we need a very narrow view of the world to survive its rigors (or if we are a Buddha) then this may suit us. In order to survive, however, we are unable to stop using the bowel altogether, although we can reduce or interfere with its function, as in anorexia nervosa. Each day we commit something of this earth to our bodies. In this way we become of the earth, or its many products, be they organically grown tomatoes or a synthetic soft drink. By the great variety of foodstuffs we select, the frequency with which we ingest them, and the process by which we choose to digest them, we indicate our love of both this planet and our body. The bowel is the organ that must continue its relationship with those things about us if we are to survive. Its place in the psychological profile of an individual is unique, and it's because of these reasons that dysfunction occurs readily in some people and why the bowel occupies such a diverse place in our body image.

The location of a bowel complaint will often indicate the area of psychological concern. Already I have indicated that lower-bowel problems are prevalent in areas of traumatic toilet training, or where an interruption of the child coming to friendly and social terms with his own excrement has occurred. Upper-bowel problems, such as gastritis, heartburn, stomach and duodenal ulcer, gallbladder problems, pancreatitis and diabetes begin in the oral-gratification stage. In this case the areas affected are those involved in the assimilation of food, rather than its excretion. People with little investment in nurturing their physical bodies will therefore be prone to upper-bowel complaints.

Needless to say, the personalities of individuals suffering from upper-intestinal complaints, or complaints of digestion, will be quite different from those suffering from complaints of excretion. Gas emanating from the upper bowel has different characteristics from that from the lower bowel, as the reaction of those unfortunate enough to be in the vicinity of the latter shows.

Food occupies such an important place in our society that I don't intend an analysis of it here. I'll do that in the section dealing with diet. I point out there that the need for instant gratification, which in Western society is breeding a generation of sugar junkies, is responsible for an enormous increase in the incidence of problems of upper-bowel assimilation, such as diabetes and hypoglycemia. Once again the physical problem (diabetes), the early childhood emotional circumstances (anxiety) and the solution to that problem (eating ice cream) have shown themselves to be interdependent. It's useless to put clients on insulin, stop them eating ice cream or treat their anxiety. All three, and usually much more, need to be considered. This takes time.

Whether for instant gratification, as in a child addicted to fruit juice, or the denial of gratification, as in an anorexic, the upper gastro-intestinal tract reflects the personality of the client. This is used by a practitioner who observes the signs, listens to the symptoms and then constructs a personality profile from this data. The early childhood decisions that the client took that resulted in both her personality and subsequently her physical symptoms are made available to the client to change using individual and group therapy techniques. A cure is effected when the client escapes the early childhood dependance on parents and subsequent parent figures, including the therapist, and takes full responsibility for herself. Within self-responsibility, I include the preparedness to make a decision to be well or unwell from a position of personal power.

THE RESPIRATORY SYSTEM

People don't get lung cancer because they smoked too many cigarettes. No, people who want to die select one of the many methods available to them that are socially acceptable at the time. Lung cancer is but one of these. The cause of a popular disease must be something that will remove the responsibility from the sufferer and "blame" an outside agent—in this case cigarettes. Now the cigarette companies, I assume, know this. When they quite rightly object to spurious data implicating cigarettes as the "cause" of lung cancer, they do so knowing that if they "conclusively proved" *no* connection between smoking and lung cancer, then the number of people smoking would quite rapidly *decrease!* Then why do they object to these falsified surveys if the proof of cigarettes as the cause of lung cancer is in their best interests? It's because they must be seen to be righteously protesting their innocence, otherwise the illusion of conspiracy and therefore "blame" is lost. If people can no longer blame cigarettes for their lung cancer, the cigarettes become redundant. There never will be any hard data on the matter because there is no such thing as hard data in the case of human beings. Statistics become meaningless. They will always show what they are required by at least one interested party to show. If one person dies of lung cancer who has not been a smoker, and of course thousands have, then smoking is not the "cause" of lung cancer. It may certainly be used to facilitate its development by those people needing to hand over their personal power to an addiction.

Those people who don't want to die of lung cancer and who want to smoke can have their cake and eat it too. If their constitution is such that they can smoke twenty cigarettes a day and withstand an obvious (self-inflicted) environmental hazard, then so be it. Smoking in this instance is clearly part of their internal balance. If I smoke more than occasionally, I have a sore throat. I am scared of some things in life and smoking is one of them. When I am really sad, scared or lonely, but am unprepared to feel those emotions, I may reach for a cigarette, play football or masturbate. When I'm less afraid, I'm prepared to feel emotions and not truncate them. Similarly, when I'm not scared, I can smoke a cigarette, enjoy it and not suffer any ill effects. There is a dynamic balance in these things. In the Orient it is called Yin and Yang. In the occident it is called Paradox.

If Father or Mother was responsible for telling the child about the dangers of smoking, and if a member of the family or a close friend died from lung cancer and that death was attributed to cigarette smoking, then heavy smoking in such an individual as a teen-ager or an adult will alert me to his existence issues, that is, his will to live. I assume that a heavy smoker with such a background has decided to not look after himself and maybe kill himself, using a method in which he was instructed in childhood. If the client smokes and genuinely does not believe it will do him any harm, then I agree with him. If he has terrible bronchitis and smokes like a train, then I assume he likes having severe bronchitis. There's no point remov-ing the bronchitis until we discover what advantages he extracts from it and how he can replace those benefits. By the time many people come to see me, they have decided that they want to change, although they may be hazy about both the old and the new sys-tem. Very few people who smoke more than twenty cigarettes a day are looking after themselves.

Sinusitis is a fascinating condition because it's so debilitating, so widespread and treated so universally badly. I have mentioned previously that it's linked with poor bowel function in most cases. The constipa-tion of the bowel reflects mental constipation, mostly in inflexible individuals, while the sinusitis (in men particularly), often indicates a reluctance to cry. The mucous membranes are chronically inflamed and swollen, a consequence of poor bowel function, envi-ronmental irritants such as pollens, exhaust fumes and cigarette smoke or a failure to be exercised and then rested appropriately. Let us examine the latter. If we're reading a book in good light, we can read easily and clearly for a time until we tire. If we then stop reading and rest our eyes, we can resume reading with no problems. However, if in poor light we continue to read beyond our capacity, we may get a headache from the strain. Instead of working properly and then resting, we have caused our eyes chronic fatigue. Mucous membranes react similarly. If we cry when we are sad, the physiological response is tears from the eyes and nose. When we've finished being sad, the mucous membranes in the nose and sinuses settle back to the normal uninflamed state. If the sadness is there but not ever directly expressed by crying (racket sadness), the mucous membranes remain chronically inflamed, never really pouring out mucus and never really resting. Low-grade inflammation results in swollen membranes that eventually block the openings to the sinuses, causing pain and further discharge. This is chronic sinusitis.

Apart from not crying effectively, the other factors contributing to the development of sinusitis are the consumption of dairy products in excess, and inadequate fiber in the diet. There are no standards. Requirements vary between individuals. Multiple allergy testing confirms what the client already knew. For this the client pays handsomely both financially and, if he ends up on the merry-go-round of desensitization treatments, physically. Usually external agents are not of much consequence in sinusitis. They can be more prominent in the causes of hay fever. When a profession has little real knowledge of an area commonly held to be within its field of expertise, spurious methods will be developed, which are recognized as useless, but which are defended aggressively by the profession for purposes of saving face. Modern medicine abounds with such spurious treatments, and might benefit from withdrawing from those areas to which doctors make little contribution and concentrating upon those in which it excels.

Upper respiratory-tract infection, the commonly designated URTI, appears on sickness certificates all over the world with a frequency probably exceeding any other illness. An URTI is a socially condoned method of taking a day or two off work. In most cases the certificate of sickness should read, "suffering from overwork, anxiety, or pique" or, more accurately, "suffering from nothing at all, but wants a rest day." To my mind it's silly for people to make themselves sick in order to take a day off work. If people were allowed to take a certain number of days without a doctor's certificate, then they could decide for themselves whether they wanted to spend the day sick in bed or whether they wanted to enjoy it. Many social systems tend to reinforce illness and discourage health.

For many people the common cold is like an old friend. For some it's their best friend or even their only friend. Rhinitis, hay fever, sore throat, tonsillitis, earache and conjunctivitis have never received recognition for the enormous amount of work that they perform in giving people days off work, getting people cared for by others, getting sympathy from lovers, avoiding unwanted appointments, confirming the world as lousy and generally providing proof of our misery for all to see. For all of these great and selfless deeds the common cold is maligned, abused, attacked with countless chemicals and even forced to undergo operations. This latter act is one of great hostility indeed and only undertaken by someone determined to appear very needy. I can imagine how this is very hurtful to the common cold, working overtime as it does with absolutely no thanks from anyone, only to be superseded in promoting non-self-responsibility by an operation. It really must be frustrating.

The common cold is not a disease so much as an institution. It is employed skilfully and effectively by those who don't want to be particulary ill but want a period of incapacity. Having achieved that incapacity they can change whatever's troubling them. Most of this is subconscious. In this way the common cold or any minor respiratory complaint is used to rebalance the psyche and the internal organs. For most people it does little long-term harm to their body but may be regarded as an unnecessary or at best inefficient way to get what they want. In addition, it's damned unpleasant! There's no point throwing it away until something equally effective and less distressing has been found to take its place. Perhaps low blood sugar (hypoglycemia) with its general incapacitation, will fulfill it's early promise.

THE CARDIO-VASCULAR SYSTEM

The client is a twenty-eight-year-old female.

"How can I help you?"
"Well, my father died of a heart attack when he was forty, my uncle died of the same thing at the age of forty-three, and my grandfather also died of a coronary when he was quite young. I'm worried that I might also die early of . . ."
"Have you any brothers?" I interrupt.
"My brother died last year of a coronary. He was thirty-two."

My face reflects the sadness I feel when anybody dies young, and my spine shivers at parental messages so dutifully and so needlessly fulfilled. The predictability, the inevitability of it. If only I could have seen him before he died, I could have guided him in deciding to live. All this is racing through my mind. I have temporarily forgotten the client's real concern with her own prognosis, but already I can tell by looking at her that the same fate won't befall her, as the family modeling was that only the men die of heart attacks. I'll return to her later.

> "What did the post-mortem show?" I inquire gently, struggling a little to conceal my interest.
>
> "There was apparently absolutely nothing to see," she replied.
>
> "What, nothing! No infarct, no coronary occlusion?"
>
> "Nothing."

I find this even more interesting, even though clients rarely give accurate pathological reports since they are rarely given accurate information.

> "What sort of man was he? Did he enjoy life, did he seem happy?"
>
> "He was a very easy-going, apparently contented, fit and healthy young man. He was an active sportsman and always had been. His diet was nothing unusual that I could see. His body was slim and muscular, and he was obviously attractive to women."
>
> "Were there any women in your family who died from heart attacks?"
>
> "There's a rumor, which my mother can't substantiate, that an old aunt of Dad's died of a heart attack, but she was quite old at the time."
>
> "Do you know that your father's, uncle's, grandfather's and brother's deaths are totally unrelated to you, as you weren't subject to the

same indoctrination in childhood that 'All of the Halisham men die young of heart attacks'?"

"Yes, that's my strong feeling and belief. I can recall talk in the family of how all the men were subject to heart attacks, and I can recall my brother being quite scared about it as a young boy, then he seemed to adjust to it and it no longer bothered him."

The interview proceeded with an explanation of the fundamentals of scripting and how diseases are passed down within families. Diet was also used as a method of reinforcing her belief that she could prevent any heart disease in herself and in her male offspring. She left with both of us feeling very confident of her good prognosis and a little sobered by the relentlessness of family dynamics.

Heart disease is interesting. Society has given it a certain significance, not unlike the niche reserved for upper-respiratory infections in community thinking. In fact, all diseases are either socially condoned or discriminated against, for very complex reasons. Popular disease is determined on anthropological criteria. I find this fascinating, because if our quest is for more pleasure and less pain, we'll need to pay some attention to our need for illness as a society.

I have discussed elsewhere how a heart attack may be precipitated when an individual is under excessive strain, often at work, and has no permission from his parents to slow down. Alternatively, part of his childhood belief system may be that in the event of overwork a heart attack is an acceptable way of confirming to himself, and demonstrating to others, that he's had enough and wants to slow down or quit. And usually, it's very effective, reserved by society as it is for just such a purpose. A man who was struggling for promotion and not enjoying it may through the good offices of a heart attack be transferred to lighter duties. The heart attack is often as effective in achieving desired changes within the family as it is at work.

Many businessmen enjoy the fight for financial security, and that's not the climate within which heart attacks are welcome. Usually they occur in dissatisfied individuals found in the more soul-destroying jobs such as production-line work than in occupations in which a person has more control over his destiny. A component of work frustration is an unwillingness to try anything different, and usually parental messages on that score were clear—parents either risked or didn't risk. Heart attacks are the result in many cases of people who have decided to work hard in order to be loved by parents, and who have no parental permission to slow down or change direction if the job no longer suits. The heart attack is condoned by the parents. Venereal disease would not serve the same purpose.

Much like the ancients, I regard the heart as the seat of the emotions. It has been fashionable in the past one-hundred years to laugh at the primitive concepts and the elementary anatomy that resulted in such an easily disproved statement. Everybody knows that the emotions reside in the brain. Well, the neurons may be firing in the brain but the physiological consequences of those emotions are reflected elsewhere, and I've already mentioned the anger that may be "stored" in the liver and the fear that affects the kidneys.

In the case of the liver, chronic anger decreases excretion of lipases, which are responsible for the absorption of fat from the diet, and may in a severe case result in chronic hepatitis. Fear may diminish blood supply to the kidneys resulting in loin pain, kidney stones or chronic kidney inflammation.

Where the heart is strong and stable, so is the personality. An individual who has a heart strongly pumping blood to all corners of the body will have visibly healthy extremeties, with beautifully sculptured hands and feet warm from the blood flow, a lively color to the skin, clear eyes, shining hair, large blood flow to the ears and vibrant genitals. I suppose I see one such person each week, and I enjoy it. They have been given the unqualified right to exist by their parents, the unhindered, uncluttered, unmodified message that they are a delight and that their existence is a joy to all. That's how they end up as adults, a delight. It's possible to teach children they can't always have their own way, and that they have an obligation to society, without modifying their right to exist. By so doing, a strong heart develops and in turn pumps health-promoting blood throughout the body. Vibrancy is the result, and it's there for all to see.

Apart from the positive aspects of a strong heart, other emotions are readily reflected by heart function. We all know that part of the "fight or flight" reaction is a rapid heart rate. When we're either scared or angry the heart rate increases and in some instances becomes irregular. Palpitations may result. Chronic sadness may result in a slow heart rate with a small output. If any of these emotions are not dealt with a small sadness (depression) or anger (aggression) may result. The long-term effect on the heart is disease.

In the case of fear, the chronic tension may result in irregularities and eventual conduction defects. Anger results in a chronically elevated cardiac output with an increase in the size of the heart muscle required to cope with the extra load. If this muscle hypertrophies (grows excessively large) beyond the capacity of its blood vessels to keep it supplied with oxygen and nutrients, or the blood vessels themselves become diseased, a heart attack results. A heart attack is simply a piece of the heart muscle dying through lack of blood. This is called an infarct. Prior to an actual heart attack, the whole cardio-vascular system may respond to an increase in blood pressure. An angry person will often have an elevated blood pressure (hypertension) prior to suffering a heart attack.

Sadness slows the heart and decreases the volume of blood (cardiac output) that it pumps to the tissues. If this continues for long enough, the tissues become undernourished and don't grow as well as they might. To see this may require close inspection. The body shape is mean, not full, the feet are cold and narrow, and the skin is dry. The person looks weak. All this may be the consequence of a mind that never believed in its right to be alive and as a consequence the heart underfunctions. People who are severely depressed are therefore physically at risk, and often die.

The cardio-vascular system, and the heart in particular, is therefore very important in the physical well-being of the individual, reflecting both his past psychological profile and his current emotional state. Games that center about illness may be played using heart disease as a pay-off to the game. With an organ as crucial to survival as the heart, these games are often played for keeps.

THE MUSCULO-SKELETAL SYSTEM

When I was a medical student and interviewing patients in hospitals, the inquiry into the musculo-skeletal system was the one I hated most. It was al-

ways so boring: arthritis, sciatica, old fractures—
hardly exciting stuff. Now that I'm older (and more
mature), I still dislike it. However, the musculo-
skeletal system is like a mirror. The other observations that I have made are often confirmed or thrown
into question after the inquiry into this system.

An individual who reports disease or injury of the
muscles, bones or joints is invariably reporting a decrease in mobility. This may be for a short time, as in
the case of a fracture, or a much longer time, as in the
increasing debilitation suffered with rheumatoid arthritis. As in all illness, if we look at the end result,
the need for the illness becomes apparent. In the case
of diseases of the skeleton, we look for the reasons the
person may benefit from a period of immobility, either
brief or protracted. Very often the immobility is
related to both physical and social withdrawal in some
form.

It's been my experience that the two features of diseases of locomotion most often present are fear and ensuing martyrdom. People who decrease their ability to
get about for any reason are usually afraid to be fully
mobile because of demands, real or imagined, that full
mobility imposes. I have noticed a high proportion of
spinsters, those women afraid to take partners, suffer
arthritis as a way of alleviating the fear of socializing
and perhaps finding a partner. I've had cases where
middle-aged women who behaved as second-class
citizens in marriages to aggressive men contracted arthritis in an effort to moderate the bullying. Others
have developed the disease to get some caring from
otherwise insensitive husbands, or have used it to
keep husbands in positions of devotion. Arthritis appears to be more common in women than in men, or
at least more debilitating, and I wonder whether
that's because in our society men prize their mobility

to a greater degree, and for them to trade immobility for the benefits of disease would be too great an imposition on their masculine self-image. Women are often less mobile anyway.

By continuing to explore arthritis in middle-aged women, I am running the risk of being labeled sexist, but most societies are sexist and sexism is one of the causes of disease. Where a woman has spent many years child-rearing, that strenuous, unpaid and often unthanked job, and where the personal rewards from seeing the children grow didn't compensate for a lack of care from her husband, she may use arthritis to confirm life as unfair, a drudge, unrewarded and long suffering. Her opinion about life is established in childhood, and for safety she deliberately picks a non-caring man to marry. He simply confirms what she already knew. A caring husband would terrify her. Martyrdom is the end result of this process, unless it's depression. I see many middle-aged women basking in the benefits of their infirmity: people, usually men, rushing to open doors; bus drivers taking longer to stop and accelerating more slowly; the hushed tones of commiseration from passers-by. The effect on others is so powerful that they would not trade their arthritis for the world. The pain, severe as it is, constitutes part of the martyrdom.

Men with arthritis, on the other hand, are generally angry. Frustrated by life, dissatisfied with work or promotion, often unloved at home, they give themselves a physical component to be angry about. This reconfirms their anger and effectively prevents them confronting other unfelt emotions, often sadness. It has been unacceptable for a man to show his sadness in our society, and as a consequence anger takes its place.

In women sadness is acceptable and anger is not. These now obsolete societal requirements have created much despair and illness.

In recent times I ruptured my Achilles tendon, which in a sportsman like myself is a serious injury, and at my age often heralds the end of a sporting career. In discussing the advantages of illness with particular reference to immobility, I believe it would be of value to look at my own case, something I was more than reluctant to do at the time. I had been back for a six-month study tour of the United States only two weeks when my old squash club called, asking me to fill in for somebody who was injured. I recall a feeling of exhilaration at being asked, as I was rather uptight at the time, and my usual method of reducing anxiety was to play competitive sport. I was fit and had been playing regularly, so there was no increased physical risk of injury. I'd been scaling down my level of aggression in sport for some years, consciously and subconsciously needing it less. This match was a return to my most aggressive style. I knew at the end of the match, waiting for me as usual would be a certain hollowness at expending all this energy and aggression, and not really getting what I wanted from it. What I wanted was love and caring but for various reasons, was at the time reluctant to secure these. My tendon snapped after I had been playing about an hour, a very close match. I recall a feeling of enormous anger, followed by sadness, which I didn't show in front of the crowd, and then the peace of "Why me?" It was a familiar question I recall from my youth, used to maintain my anger at parents who didn't give me what I wanted. Instead of asking directly, I justified my fear and anger by claiming fate, not I, was responsible.

The injury required surgical repair, I was in a cast for several months and have been inactive for the pastyear, a considerable imposition. I believe that I'll fully recover. Next time when I want some caring, I'll ask for it, or if I'm afraid to do that, I'll do something that takes care of me and is safe.

A history of repeated fractures indicates either a constitution lacking in essential minerals, or a person who "likes" being injured. The latter is almost always the case, and if an individual reports frequent vehicular accidents, recalled with great excitement, I consider that he's trying to kill himself and look for a "don't exist" injunction from one or both parents. In the case of youths riding motorbikes, there's often little willingness to acknowledge the fact that death is final, as group prestige is gauged by willingness to defy death. I believe that nearly all "accidents" are engineered by the subconscious. I hesitate to say "there's no such thing as an 'accident,' " preferring to believe that there's no such thing as "no such thing." The distinction, as we will see later, is important.

Back pain is one of the most frequent complaints with which a general practitioner is confronted. It may well be of an acute nature and be the presenting complaint, but in a detailed history that invites listing all problems is more often squeezed in at the end. As such it represents one of life's little obstacles, one of those irritations about which Englishmen have been heard to mumble with resignation, "Mustn't grumble." Unlike my early days when I followed my teaching, which was that you basically ignored it and it went away, or the patient at least stopped complaining to you about it, I take careful note of back pain as it's a very helpful indicator of the progress a client's making in therapy. If a client decides to resolve those issues that have been contributing to her illness, then back pain usually disappears without fanfare.

"By the way, Mrs. Bonkowski, how's your back pain you told me about when you first came two months ago?"

"To tell the truth, Doctor, I had completely forgotten about it. Yes, isn't that amazing, it'd been there for years!"

I gave her no active treatment for an extremely irritating complaint and it nevertheless disappeared. She subconsciously decided to drop it.

Causes of back pain and the reasons they respond to psychotherapy are too numerous to list. Back pain, I have said, is a good indicator of progress. When a client remakes some decisions about her life and changes direction, those decisions are often accompanied by some dramatic changes to her physical appearance. The individual may stand up so much straighter than before that she grows an inch in height, or walk with a new spring in her step, which alters the back tensions and posture. The stoop of depression may be lost, or excessive weight may be shed. All of these things dramatically alter back pain. I have found this previously chronically frustrating area of practice to be very rewarding using this style of alternative medicine.

I have briefly discussed, using the shape of the diagnostic frame, those areas of the psychological profile contributing to the illness. We'll await the physical examination to evaluate it further.

THE GENITO-URINARY SYSTEM

Sex plays a large part in the life of human beings and has often been exploited by those prepared to maintain power over others using guilt, for example, the church. Diseases of the genito-urinary system reflect this.

Sex may be flirtatious, esoteric, intimate, aggressive, casual, wild and passionate, passive, fast, noisy, tantalizing, dominant, rhythmical, elusive, slow, quiet, fulfilling or disappointing. It may be regular, frequent or rare. It may be a way of life, a way to deny closeness and caring, the icing on a wholesome cake, a reason to adopt a radical political or religious viewpoint, an effective method of maintaining guilt, or a self-pleasuring activity. It may occupy an individual totally or not at all. It may be an act of love of both self and others, or an act of hostility, intended to hurt both parties. Anything capable of such great pleasure and love must be capable of the antitheses of those things, according to the law of Yin and Yang, or the law of Eternal Change. Night and day, heat and cold, fast and slow all move imperceptibly from one into the other. There is no single point where one stops and the other starts. They are all part of the same continuum. The sexually permissive person is often similar to the sexually outraged one who sees sex as the scourge of the earth, and would have all offenders whipped. Despite apparently diametrically opposed behaviors, the psychological position may be similar (see diagram on page 200). For the child, sex and punishment are often linked. Use and abuse, excess and denial are all part of the cyclical nature of our sexualities, individually and collectively as a society. We use sex to sell things and as a consequence are assailed by it relentlessly. It's one of the last free pleasures, and a part of us that we can deny but not ignore. Only a person with no eyes and ears may escape people and things being advertised using sex, and then such an individual would be so refreshingly naive that to some she would anyway be considered a prized sexual object. Innocence would rapidly be lost. In this climate of active sexuality, it's

Finding the Cause

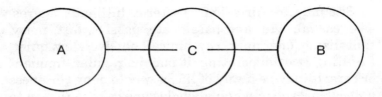

The linear notion of the spectrum of opinions

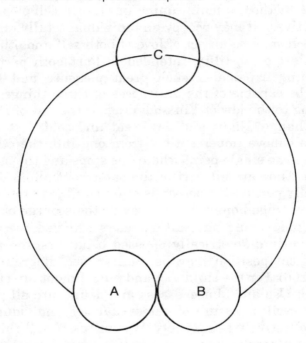

The continuum of opinions

A. Sex is everything.
B. Sex is sinful.
C. Sex is what you make it.

Using the circular concept, it is evident that the two strident positions are actually the closest despite protesting themselves to be polar opposites. The please-yourself option remains neutral in both models.

no wonder that sex is considered a large part of the personality, and equally no wonder that our body image is dominated by our sexuality. Because of these things, diseases of the genito-urinary system constitute a significant proportion of current medical practice, and like all diseases, indicate the relevant area of the client's psyche.

For years my own preference was to deny closeness in favor of sexual promiscuity. By so doing I felt safe. This personal characteristic is potentially both a gold mine and a pitfall in my effectiveness as a therapist. On the positive side, I'm able to identify a sexual nuance, either expressed or denied, readily, and this is very effective in establishing why a man should be suffering from herpes or a woman is unable to conceive. Equally helpful is the fact that I'm not afraid of my own sexuality, and I give clients permission to have their own sexual feelings. I'm happy to show a middle-aged matron how to masturbate, pointing out the clitoris and discussing those methods that women who masturbate report as being pleasurable. I am equally at ease with the concern a middle-aged man shows for his future sex life following a diagnosis of prostatism and happy to comment favorably upon the erection a youth has sustained during examination, rather than pretending it didn't happen.

Often I'm the first person with whom a middle-aged woman has ever discussed masturbation and orgasm. It's remarkable to me how freely these women are prepared to speak of such matters, coming from a generation that was taught that any concern with sex was unbecoming in a woman. As I'm the age of the sons of these women, my surprise is probably more a reflection of the way I conceived mothers as sexless beings than anything else. Any personal bias of mine is capable of distorting my therapy, if I'm unaware of it. In any event, when given the chance, people who haven't spoken of their sexuality for years, or at all, usually have a few questions stored up. They express relief at the chance to discuss things that have long bothered them.

All of this is possible if the practitioner allows people the time and provides the climate in which it's safe to express feelings. Of course, some women will react adversely if questioned about sexual function and that's equally as informative as the answers they might have given.

With young people, I'm careful to assess their state of maturity before taking a sexual history. A large proportion of sixteen-year-olds have had intercourse, and for them questions dealing with sex and masturbation are usually not problematical. Between ten and fifteen, teenagers are at various stages of awakening sexuality and I'm careful to respect that. I have known a ten-year-old boy to be having regular intercourse with his twelve-year-old neighbor over a two-year period. This was no problem for either of them—obviously they enjoyed it—and my guess is once the novelty has worn off they will be ambivalent about sex until a further awakening later in their teens. For their parents it was more of an ordeal but, much to their credit, both defined the problem as their own, at the same time wanting to protect their children. At the ages of ten and twelve, children in this society still want parental direction and protection.

One of the more insidious aspects of current orthodox medical practice is the way in which doctors make a lot of money and a lot of mistakes in the area of women's problems. Problems of contraception, menarche, menopause, menstruation, conception, urinary tract infections, vaginal infections and sexual disinterest constitute a large proportion of the average doctor's practice. There's no evidence that female doctors counsel women any more effectively than their male colleagues in these areas, though to be sure their experience is first hand and women often feel more comfortable during the physical examination if the doctor is female. Whereas male practitioners may dismiss female complaints with scorn, derision or simple disbelief accompanying unresolved grudges towards their own mothers, a woman doctor on the other hand may, by joining in a game of "Ain't it awful" with the client, contribute to her misconception of the disease as not of her own making. The refusal of doctors of both sexes to make themselves aware of the sexual games they are playing in their own lives prevents accurate diagnosis and effective treatment of their client's problem. Because there's considerable polarization of the sexes, there's also considerable distrust.

In general terms, people who enjoy their own sexuality will not suffer from diseases of the sexual organs. Alternatively, an individual who comes to rely upon his sexuality for intimacy, to the exclusion of friendship, can expect that if he's unhappy a disturbance of his genitals will be made more likely. The source of comfort becomes a source of frustration, and if a man translates this into self-hate, a disease of the genitals confirms to him that he's unworthy. In the case of a man who's become sexually promiscuous from rebelling against his puritanical mother, developing cancer of the penis merely highlights his failure to discard the old belief system. The following case is such an example.

Jeff Peters was a thirty-three-year-old man who came to see me with a diagnosis of cancer of the testicle. The right testicle had been removed at operation and his prognosis was good. He wanted to learn how to avoid the chain of events contributing to his disease, and thereby prevent a recurrence.

He had had an unhappy childhood, being the only son of parents who had fought a protracted divorce, an event he recalled as being extremely traumatic. His mother, with whom he'd lived following the departure of his father, had often said that her only reason for living was to be with him. Without him, life wasn't worth living. She exhorted him to never leave her and would sabotage the romantic affairs he began as a teenager and young man by becoming distraught with the idea that one day he'd get married and abandon her. As a consequence, he related poorly to women and had never established a satisfactory relationship.

When he was twenty-nine, he and his mother took a brief excursion to a neighboring town, a distance of some fifty kilometers. On the return journey, he rolled their car and his mother was killed. He blamed himself for the accident and, having been very angry at his mother for the ruthless way in which she attempted to dictate his life, felt very guilty that subconsciously he'd wanted to kill her. This was no doubt the case, and the normal reaction of a child to parents who aren't providing what he wants by way of love and protection. Two years after the accident, when he'd been in a promising relationship with a woman for a year, he developed cancer of the testis. He reported that he still dwelt on both the accident and his mother's plea to "never marry a woman and leave me." He knew he was giving himself a serious illness in order to atone for both these sins. The one he'd chosen, threatening both his sexuality and his life, was quite specific. No other would have done.

For a number of reasons I sent him to another therapist. He became sufficiently aware of the dynamics of his illness to decide to both live and feel good about his sexuality. For him, that is wellness. Wellness includes both awareness and the willingness to take responsibility for decisions we make in our best interests. It does not necessarily mean the absence of disease but rather taking responsibility for those diseases we decide to have.

Most women have suffered from painful periods at some stage in their lives. If the pain is severe, then analgesia is required. Occasional disturbances will be a reaction to stress, pollutants, not wanting to have sex, fluid retention or many other factors. Provided pain is not a regular event, then beyond the inconvenience the disturbance is of little consequence. If painful periods (dysmenorrhea), excessive blood loss (menorrhagia), decreased blood flow (oligomenorrhea), absent periods (amenorrhea) or any other disturbance of menstruation is regular, answers to how these problems have arisen will be found with great regularity in the area of the woman's sexuality.

For an organ or a body system to be healthy, it requires a certain amount of exercise. If it is underexercised, then it runs the risk of deterioration, through diminished blood supply. If overused, it may hypertrophy and run out of blood supply, become exhausted, or create imbalances elsewhere. In both cases, malfunction of that organ or system results, and is followed by embarrassment to others, which are then forced to compensate for the increased or decreased function of the aberrant system. The lungs, for example, may be required to handle a greater acid load as a consequence of temporary shutdown of the kidneys.

The kidneys, in turn, may be forced to handle a greater solid load as a consequence of the failure of an enzyme system. This may result in gout. Many systems, the liver, pancreas, thyroid and adrenals, may be overworking in order to compensate for a great overuse of the gut during an eating binge. Let's apply these principles to the genito-urinary system.

A woman who enjoys her sexuality, loves her body, admires her breasts and finds looking at her genitals a pleasurable experience will generally be guaranteeing their well-being. If, in addition, she enjoys having her naked body admired by others and enjoys having regular intercourse with one or more partners, frequently experiencing orgasm or fulfillment without guilt, she will have healthy sexual organs. The frequency of sexual contact will, of course, vary tremendously, and one is no more desirable than the other. For health, the requirements are simply that enough regular blood flow be established to keep the part active, and that the woman regard her body and sexuality as things of great beauty. By so doing, the clitoris will be sensitive, the vagina will be well lubricated and relaxed, the cervix will have a healthy blood flow capable of being buffeted by the penis during intercourse, and the womb will contract, build up and empty with efficiency and minimal discomfort. The woman's self-image as a fertile, sexually responsive person will guarantee a regular, effective ovulation, often synchronized to either the cycle of the moon or another woman with whom she has an intimate relationship, or with whom she shares a house. Regular, trouble-free menstruation, with an absence of ovarian problems, results. Conception is effortlessly achieved when the woman decides she's ready to have a baby. That decision will need to be both subconscious and conscious, otherwise pregnancy will not result.

Conditioning with regard to childbirth and child-rearing is usually powerful, and at the time the woman considers having a baby all these early childhood stories resurface. If they are mainly frightening, they may well upset ovulation and render the woman temporarily infertile. The period of infertility may last from between a few months to the whole of her child-rearing years. It depends on how soon she resolves the fears, and that usually depends on how great those fears are.

If a mother repeatedly tells her daughter she nearly died giving birth, the girl is likely to decide at an early age that childbirth is dangerous and to be avoided. There are, of course, other causes of infertility that are less directly related to the mind, such as diet, drug addiction, congenital deformities of the genital tract, past infections of the ovarian tubes and hormonal irregularities. It's my belief that the large percentage of infertile women who have been investigated and who demonstrate no obvious physiological or anatomical pathology have decided to remain infertile.

If you ask "What's frightening about being pregnant?" and the answer "Nothing!" is snapped back at you, you have confirmed the presence of underlying fear. Psychotherapy helps the woman resolve the fear of pregnancy, and a child results. Men, of course, are often responsible for the failure of a couple to produce offspring, and I believe their case histories affect fertility. If we look at a couple of examples of women preventing themselves from conceiving, the psychological mechanisms become clearer.

Melissa came to see me when she was thirty, complaining of a failure to conceive. She'd been married for about eight years and her husband had always wanted children. She was more wary. The gynecologists and obstetricians had given her a clean bill of health. Her problem in orthodox terms was a failure to ovulate, something that had been difficult to remedy with the drugs available for that purpose. Her husband had a normal sperm count. She believed that for one or more reasons she was preventing herself becoming pregnant.

She was an exceptionally attractive woman with beautiful big eyes, a very handsome face and a slim figure that she dressed to perfection. She flirted with me and I with her. She had obviously learned early in life that she was attractive to men, and in fact reported that her father loved her so dearly that her mother was jealous. Mother and father had expended their relationship by the time Melissa was born and had lapsed into an uneasy truce. Melissa became the number one girl in her father's life and he would say so quite unashamedly. She enjoyed this favored position, even though her mother reacted with anger at being rejected by her husband in favor of her daughter and took out her frustrations by being sarcastic to Melissa. Melissa believed fathers had daughters in favor of whom they abandoned their wives. This made their wives very unhappy.

Melissa was now the wife. If she had a daughter by her child-adoring husband, chances were that he would abandon her. This is what she'd experienced in childhood and there was no reason to suspect that things were any different now. She wasn't prepared to risk her marriage for a child. In addition, her mother had blamed the arrival of the children for her own miserable existence, and had stated frequently that "children tie you down and force you into intolerable situations." This was hardly an encouraging reflection. No, having children was definitely not in Melissa's best interests.

Therapy involved her deciding that she hadn't married her father, and receiving assurances from her husband that he wouldn't abandon her when the baby was born. In addition, she realized that if things didn't work out between them she could always leave. Her body changed significantly over a period of six months. The somewhat girlish figure was replaced by a much fuller womanly sensuality, the type one associates with women who enjoy their own sexuality immensely. She decided to postpone having a baby until she felt safer about it and, as a final twist to the story, began practicing contraception after "trying" all those years to become pregnant. Where a woman has not become pregnant and over the years has not used contraception, believing herself from experience to be infertile, the commencement of contraception is a clear indication that she is now approaching fertility. If she reports that, "I've never bothered with contraception and I've never been pregnant but I thought I'd better stop taking risks," I assume she's decided that she'll start ovulating. Melissa has now conceived.

Nor do I exclude men with low sperm counts from the responsiblity of being unable to father children. I believe that male infertility is just as responsive to psychological factors as a woman's failure to ovulate. I'm unable to prove this, as I don't have any experience with men with low sperm counts over a long period of time, but there's no acceptable proof in such matters anyway.

If women or girls complain of small breasts, or if men or boys complain of a small penis, I'm interested in how that's a problem for them. I don't accept the opinion of the client as necessarily borne out by the physical examination. What we are dealing with here is a problem of body image. If a woman has small breasts then I presume she needed small breasts for some reason and I wonder, now that she has them, why she should give herself a hard time over them. If I can establish why she needs to criticize herself, and why she's chosen the size of her breasts to effect this, it may be unnecessary to change the breasts themselves. She may end up delighted with her small breasts. If she decides she no longer needs the small breasts, she will allow her hormonal systems to enlarge them. As breasts are involved in both sexual attraction and in child-feeding, it may be safely assumed that the poor body image revolves about issues to do with either or both of these things.

A fifteen-year-old boy came to see me a year ago complaining about his small penis. At his insistence, his mother waited in the waiting room during the interview. It was clear that there was some sexual injunction from the mother toward her son's sexuality, and much to her credit she had realized this; she brought him to me. He was grossly obese for a fifteen-year-old, a time when boys are often letting their manhood flower in the form of fine muscles and a proud posture. His penis wasn't visible from beneath the pudendal fat, and I thought at first that he was not exaggerating his problem. After speaking with him for some time, I invited him to stroke his penis and, if he felt safe, get an erection. Such parental permission is rarely forthcoming. He did this willingly and immediately sustained a large erection that was more than one would expect of a young teenager. Clearly there was nothing wrong with his penis, and he had kept himself fat to hide his sexuality. I suggested he go away and masturbate, which he was doing already, and not feel guilty about it. When I saw him after six months, he was much slimmer and no longer had a problem with the size of his penis. I believe that men who have a genuinely small penis can alter the size to some degree by psychotherapy. I have no experience of this but am led to conclude it from the other physical changes I've seen people make.

Herpes is one of the curses of our time. Unfortunately, I don't have a cure for it. I've tried just about everything that has appeared remotely encouraging in both the medical and lay literature, all with little success. I haven't been able to attribute those few successes I have had to the particular remedy in question. Homeopathic remedies for a time seemed valuable in herpes of the lip, but not in genital herpes. The condition is incredibly widespread and probably increasing. The literature is full of the suffering that clients experience as a consequence of such a serious disturbance of their sexual functioning, but my perpective is that it's their sexual attitudes that have resulted in the herpes, not the other way round.

At the time of contracting the disease they have needed to modify their sexuality or have a "need" to be miserable or appear to be the victim of fate. None of us, it seems, likes to see ourselves as totally responsible for ourselves, and for the purpose of proving that we're the victims of circumstance to some degree, are prepared to give ourselves illnesses. This reaffirms our vulnerability. Under pressure we tend to revert to the relative safety of childhood beliefs and practices.

A condition like herpes which has such a disturbing effect on a person's sexuality must reflect his attitude to his own sexuality in general, and his genitals in particular. If children are taught that all parts of their bodies are both wonderful and to be respected, and that the feelings they get from them are welcome and healthy, I believe they're less likely to suffer from genital herpes than someone who has been fed the usual garbage that sex is unclean, that you mustn't touch yourself in those areas and that "nice girls don't." The prevalence of genital herpes reflects the prevalence in our society of some very bigoted and powerful sexual conditioning. This is in contrast to the belief of some religious and "moral" organizations, which in the hope of achieving conversions, propagate their own sexual pathology, that is, that sexual diseases are caused by too much sex in the community. They are in fact the result of too many parental injunctions about sex. If parents encouraged their children to find their own style of sexual fulfillment, the matter would defuse. People would be uninterested in the sexual habits of their neighbors. In such a climate, sexual disturbances, which are the end result of parental and societal bigotry, would disappear, as would herpes and other diseases of the sex organs.

I've treated a few cases of genital herpes in great depth by group psychotherapy over a period of a year, and while I can report a decrease in the frequency and severity of attacks, I cannot report a cure. The fringe benefits are, however, worth the exercise alone, or so my clients report. If a pill or vaccination is developed to cure genital herpes, at this stage I would recommend taking the pill and changing the sexual injunctions later.

Before we leave the topic of sexuality, there's a final point that should be made. As a society, we are more concerned with sex and money than perhaps with anything else. Both of these things can be and are used to create divisions within the society. I do not think that this is wittingly orchestrated by any particular political lobby, although it's certainly in the interests of big business to keep people to some degree separate, and in small and numerous buying units, that is, couples or families. Additionally, it's probably in the best interests of politicians generally, as they are clearly of the belief that they know what's best for all, to discourage any closeness between people that might generate independence. My point is that factors are operating in the community to keep people away from each other, scared of each other, distrusting and skeptical of each other, and that these attitudes are promoted by interested parties. What has this got to do with the diseases of the genito-urinary tract?

Sex and closeness are two of many variables that in any relationship constantly change. On one end of the sexual spectrum may be the classic "Wham, bam, thank you, Ma'am," and on the other, long-term, nonsexual friendship. There is not a thing wrong with either contact. If either is practiced to the exclusion of the other, however, imbalance results, and disease follows imbalance.

Many people practice a combination of the above types of personal interaction and are satisfied by the arrangement. If they have a monogamy contract with their spouse, they may allow their casual sexual drives to be satisfied by flirting. Given the emphasis on sexuality in the community and the lack of closeness, however, many people in fact use their sexuality to avoid getting close to other people. This attitude is actively promoted by some churches and by others who preach that sex is bad, thereby encouraging anyone indulging to feel bad about it and to withdraw for his crimes. With the media at every opportunity encouraging people to have sex, and the prevailing moral overtone that it's a sin (hence it is hidden from parents, teachers and others), the climate for casual sex is established.

People often end up with frequent sexual contact and no real caring, and that's imbalance. Those who actively campaign against sex are of course achieving the opposite result from that which they intended.

An alternative attitude would be to allow children whatever sexual contact they liked, and teach them ways to assess the caring available to them to both receive and to give in the relationship. They could also be taught to look for signs that indicate danger. Very soon people would be establishing sexual contacts with people who cared as well. By doing these things, sexuality would disappear as a contentious issue, making many people's lives so much more fulfilling and guilt free, and the major predisposition towards sexual diseases would be removed. Sowing the seeds of health in children is *real* preventive medicine.

THE CENTRAL NERVOUS SYSTEM— AWARENESS VS. ASPIRIN

Diseases of the brain and spinal cord are afforded considerable status in medicine. They are considered somewhat exotic and the practitioners who deal with them, neurologists and neurosurgeons, occupy an exalted position in the medical hierarchy. Diseases of these systems therefore appeal to a certain type of patient, particularly medical practitioners. You can almost hear the little kid doctor in them saying, "Nah, nah, my disease beats your disease!" Many of the diseases of the nervous system are considered incurable, like multiple sclerosis, neurofibromatosis, Huntington's chorea and trigeminal neuralgia, so people don't have to give them up after they've spent time and effort in establishing them. If they decide on a tumor of the brain, the neurosurgical team may operate for fifteen hours, sometimes successfully, and the follow-up treatment is usually the best the hospital can provide. Diseases of the central nervous system are truly the doyens of diseases.

I don't know whether the common headache is the most commonly experienced discomfort or dis-ease in humans, but it must be close. It's important as well because I think that it represents the area where most people will allow themselves to look a little more closely at the circumstances of their feeling unwell. Whereas few people will admit any role in the development of their arthritis, and no one will admit to contributing to their multiple sclerosis, most people will admit to tension or aggravations at work or home as features of recurrent headaches. That's a start and you have to start somewhere.

> "How can I change my life so that I can stop having these headaches and not have to take these pills?"
> "What must I do to learn to relax?"

Headaches are used to avoid so many things that if you suffer headaches and want to find out why, look at the end result of having them. For example, if a headache at home means your wife stops talking about the neighbor's problems, ask yourself whether you aren't sick of hearing about others' problems. If you take time off work with headaches, ask yourself if you really want that job. If you suffer from headaches after intercourse, ask yourself what you're feeling and what you're saying about yourself having had intercourse, and you will establish a benefit from that feeling or thought.

Of course, some people turn head pain into life-threatening illnesses such as brain cancer, and occasionally some of these people decide that they don't want to die after all and survive, often with the help of the neurosurgeons. Each person suffering headaches must decide for himself how much he wants the condition investigated because he's the only person who really knows how much self-harm he's capable of. Therein lies the great flexibility of the headache. It can be used to manipulate a marriage for years (with the approval of both parties of course), or can be an occasional thing, reserved perhaps for avoiding weddings.

The frequency, severity and the area of application of the headache are often taught quite specifically in childhood, since the very real hard work of caring for children is one of the tasks capable of being moderated by a headache. By protesting that she has a headache, a mother may entice a reluctant husband to wash the dishes, for example. Children therefore learn about these things early. Boys may learn that if they come home late from the bar and claim a headache, then they feel better about the severe admonishing they have courted and consequent expiation of their guilt, whereas girls may learn that instead of being angry at your husband, you give yourself a headache, seduce him and then claim insensitivity on his part. Both parties have predictably (and in these examples stereotypically) given up their own power and self-responsibility in favor of having a headache. It seems almost a silly thing to do, given an outcome where both partners remain secretly angry at each other and neither is satisfied, but that simply demonstrates the power of the early conditioning. A child who has experienced the manipulation possible with skillful use of the headache is clearly going to believe that illness is an acceptable way of relating to loved ones. The likelihood is that she'll use similar tactics, or be so outraged at the dishonesty that she'll rebel and never suffer from headaches. If she is rebelling as an adult and still angry at her parents, she will most likely choose another form of incapacitation, perhaps recurrent laryngitis. You'll hear her protest that, "At least I never suffered from headaches!" If she gets mad as hell at her parents for what she didn't get, and for the sham she witnessed, understands that they were doing what was safest for them in threatening circumstances, and drops the anger, she's unlikely to need anything of significance to be wrong with her. I repeat the basis of this thesis: *If you have no need of major illness, you will have no major illness.*

Everything that we become aware of as children or adults must register through one or more of the five sensory channels: sight, sound, touch, smell and taste. We experience things through these channels, and when we recall the events of childhood, it's likely that the recollection will favor one or more senses above the others. In such a way the smell of a gasoline truck passing may be a more vivid memory than the sound. It is for me. Some people will regularly favor one system of registering events, so that a person may be identifiable as a visual person, an auditory person, a kinesthetic person (one who registers movement) or as an olfactory person. The system primarily used by the individual is known as his representational system— see S. R. Lankton, *Practical Magic*, Meta Publications, California, 1980. The particular system favored by the individual will be evident in his language, for example, "I can see you don't believe me," is the way in which a visual person may speak. An auditory person may say, "It's obvious that you don't believe what I'm saying!" while an olfactory person may say, "Well, the whole thing *smells* of insincerity!" To communicate effectively with people, it's helpful to be in the same representational system as they are. Hypnosis makes use of the sensory preference of the subject in just this way.

In considering diseases of the central nervous system, we are obliged to consider diseases of the sense organs, such as blindness, deafness, loss of taste and various sensory defects. Some sensory aberrations are in fact diseases of the peripheral nervous system, and some diseases such as tertiary syphilis affect both the central and peripheral nervous systems. The defect in the ability of the sense organ to register events taking place about it varies from minor to complete, for example, from a minor visual defect to total loss of sight. Many of these defects, particularly the severe ones, are present at birth and are a consequence of genetics, poor diet or lifestyle of the parents, environmental pollutants such as lead from car exhausts, or infections such as rubella. Most are avoidable, some are not. Those that develop later, often in childhood or as a young adult, may be the consequence of making a decision to shut down the function of that organ. That decision is nearly always subconscious. Someone with no obvious physical trauma can suddenly, or over a period of time, no longer see. Another individual may slowly lose hearing until he is partially or completely deaf. The hearing loss may be a nerve-conduction defect and in some cases be accompanied by tinnitus (ringing in the ear). There often appears to be no logical explanation for the onset or the continuation of the disease. Under those circumstances I ask myself (and then the client) what it is that's too frightening for the client to either see or hear. What's so terrifying for them that the safest way out is to simply not register events around them?

It may be an acute thing, like not wanting to hear

what the boss says at work, and then claiming compensation for industrial hearing loss. Or it may be chronic, deep-seated anxiety, as in the case of the orphan who was told by her stepmother that she was only given a home because of her poor sight. Recovering sight to this girl may well have meant a loss of support. Until she feels safe enough to take care of herself, which may be never, she'll keep the visual defect. She'll marry a man who feels so inadequate that he needs to atone for his unworthiness by looking after someone full-time. Such men will often choose as partners people who want to remain in need of care and who, in order to justify this arrangement continuing, cite their sensory disability.

Now if I were suffering from a major hearing or sight loss of inexplicable origin and I were reading this, I might have one of two reactions. Firstly, I could be absolutely outraged and shout something like, "What the hell would he know anyway!" and retreat into my private but not very helpful explanation of the disease, or I could say, "Well, I don't know, but neither does anybody else, it may help. I'll ask myself a few questions about it and see if I can't establish my investment, if any in this disability." The first approach won't yield results right now because the individual is still protecting himself. That's the best thing for him to do at this point, enjoy his outrage. In the future he may feel safe enough to think about it. The second option establishes the benefits, if any, of the disease and may or may not be helpful at this time. The pathology may be so longstanding as to be irreversible but, on the other hand, real gains may be made. The power exercised in the creation of the problem is harnessed to remove it. This will be both frightening and exciting. The prize and the risk will always be balanced.

10

Drugs, Diet and Personality— Who's Taking What?

MEDICATION

In Australia approximately 55 percent of people take regular medication of some description in any two weeks, as noted earlier, on page 152. Of those drugs taken, about 50 percent are prescribed by a medical practitioner, the rest are prescribed by naturopaths or bought in supermarkets or health food shops. These figures are staggering, demonstrating that a majority of the population believes in taking drugs frequently. When the drugs of social intercourse are included, nicotine from tobacco, caffeine from tea and coffee, and alcohol, it becomes clear that most people living in developed nations are under the influence of drugs all, or most, of their lives. Think about it for a moment, and see if that applies to you. What would life be like for you if you couldn't take drugs?

Why do so many people take so much medication? I believe it's simply an end result of being afraid to take full responsibility for ourselves.

Several drugs have been developed, which have dramatically altered the course of disease for some people, if not saved their lives. Penicillin, insulin and cortisone come to mind, and if we add aspirin, morphine, digoxin and the "pill," drugs that have affected the quality of life, we have almost assembled the significant advances in medicine over the past fifty years. Following the Second World War, people were led to believe that along with the great social reconstructions and burgeoning affluence, health and longevity were problems capable of being solved by technology. The enormous quantity of drugs consumed by the community is a legacy of that belief. Psychologically, the consumption of drugs is synonymous with administering happiness. "If you take this pill you'll feel better (and all your troubles will go away)."

Becoming materialistic and affluent has bred its own share of new social and emotional problems, and so has the belief in the theory of instantaneous drug cure. We hoped, quite reasonably, that it would work. We hoped that while the politicans and the capitalists or the totalitarian regimes would make us happy and prosperous, the doctors would make us well. I'm sorry to inform you that the experiment has failed. I'm sorry to inform you that for the large majority of people, drugs, in the long term, make things worse. I am sorry to inform you that you must, if you wish to be well, look after yourself. When I say I'm sorry, I mean that I am sorry for me: sorry that a parent won't look after me for the rest of my life, sorry that they will not do it and did not do it perfectly when they had the chance. By taking pills, we are assuming the inventor, discoverer, manufacturer, prescriber and dispenser all know more about us than we do, and that in their collective wisdom, they will take care for us. Taking the drug, I have said, is like taking "happiness." It represents the parent that we hoped, like Buddha or Jesus Christ, would make us secure, loved and happy. I'm not admonishing you in this, I'm commiserating with you. This crisis consists of both danger and opportunity. The danger is of deciding to remain loveless, helpless, hopeless and ill, and the opportunity is to take full responsibility for ourselves and to harness the power within. That way we will be our own parent, our own physician, and have little need for drugs.

The frequency and the nature of the remedies taken by clients helps me understand how much they have relied upon orthodox or unorthodox remedy, folk remedy, family remedy, or self-administration to keep themselves well. Conversely, taking people off medication is like prying a bone from the jaws of a hungry dog—not to be undertaken lightly. The medication is often an integral part of the client's belief system, and a rapid change may be too frightening for him and counterproductive. I found that out through being bitten a few times. My practice was to insist that the client immediately stop taking all medication. Now I wean people off medication only after they have established ways of caring for themselves. If they are "a pack of nerves," they'll be taking a pack of tranquilizers (presumably one for each nerve), or if they are too scared to be diagnosed as ill but feel lousy, they may be on twenty vitamins a day. Usually this makes them feel nauseous but at least they are looking after themselves. If they're a bit trendy, and enjoy the game of "My doctor out-diagnoses your doctor," then homeopathy, with its appreciation of idiosyncrasy and personal prescription, will probably be the choice. Doctors' daughters who were abandoned by their fathers at the appearance of their first pubic hair or breast bud, and who subsequently never forgave their fathers for not continuing to touch them, may be rebelliously taking no medication at all. They'll boom it out at you, the anger scarcely concealed, "I never take drugs of any description!" I may get them taking some drug as a way of energizing their impasse.

The role of drugs in contemporary society is complex and concerned not only with people's needs but also with big business, power, money and technology. Drug companies are among the most powerful institutions on earth.

SOCIAL HISTORY

This section is perhaps the most significant in the history because it's the place I confirm previous observations, or make adjustments where I have been incomplete or wrong. I believe that the psychological profile of any person and her body must be consistent, that is, they must mutually reflect what is happening in each other. The same can be said of a client's personal circumstances. Events in an individual's life that are normally considered to be totally unrelated to her medical state are in fact reflective of her physical state, and vice versa. Hence, personal circumstances reflect both the psychological and physical state. Life events that are never the subject of medical inquiry are in fact just as informative as an orthodox history, and far more informative than the vast majority of laboratory tests. People who are generally happy are generally well. I don't believe that illness "causes" unhappiness any more than I believe that unhappiness "causes" illness. Unhappiness and illness are states of mind, *reactions* to events and are at once mutually supportive, mutually antagonistic and constantly changing. This paradigm will emerge as the corner-stone of both the understanding of illness and, more particularly, its treatment. Let us consider an example. (I had acne myself, so this example, like the rest of this theory, is close to my heart.) If a boy has acne, and he uses this to remind himself of how ugly he is, the acne "causes" him to be unhappy. But the acne developed because he was unhappy about the way he looked. He increased the secretions of his sebaceous glands, using hormonal control, and the muscular tension in his face closed off the pores, resulting in acne. Therefore, the unhappiness "causes" the acne. This example demonstrates *mutual support* between unhappiness and acne. The boy, however, is happy to have his opinion about his looks confirmed by the acne (illness "causes" happiness) and, in turn, is content to be unhappy (unhappiness "causes" wellness) because at the moment that is safest for him. In this context, being well means taking care of greater fears. The same example has now demonstrated *mutual antagonism*. When this boy matures and drops some of his fears about being attractive and wants to attract admirers we can expect him to gradually remove his acne. The relationship between his illness and his happiness will then be different and will continue to fluctuate over the years, that is, it will be *constantly changing*.

I have never seen an unattractive person who did not "want" to be unattractive. The psyche has, over a period of time, faithfully sculptured the bones, muscles and skin to suit the individual. Additionally, belief in self-beauty always transcends those asymmetrical facial features caused by genetics or old misadventure. Social circumstances may be used both to determine causes and plan treatment programs for illness. Self-love, the fabric of both love for others and wellness, is evident in the everyday life of an individual.

Happy people are healthier than unhappy people. That's a bold statement, which you may confirm by thinking of yourself or others that you know who were ill, and remembering the events in your lives at the time. The personal circumstances of individuals will reflect their medical history, and vice versa. As I have said earlier, one does not "cause" the other. The social environment at any time, like the physical state, is a reflection of the early life decisions that were taken as a child. That's why the social history is of such value. It will often verify that clients are not getting what they want for themselves in their lives and, in these circumstances, it's unlikely the client is protecting himself from physical disease.

We all know people who appeared to be very happy in their personal life, perhaps happily married with lovely kids, a good income, a nice home, were well respected, good looking and in the prime of their life who have been stricken by a serious illness and maybe died. How does that fit into the theory of personal circumstances correlating with illness? We all know as well of people who appeared to have all those advantages and who turn out to be less than we thought. I say "less," because it's a feature of all of us, in our quest for someone, somewhere, to look after us, or to be a higher authority than we are, that we readily hoist others onto pedestals and are then shocked when they don't turn out as we fantasized, for our own needs, they would. Once again, we are angry at having been betrayed, or at least not looked after properly, by our parents. No one is a higher authority on you than you are. (You can still pick the brains of whoever makes himself available to help you.)

Firstly, our impression of the "beautiful people" who have "got it all together," and who, as a consequence, should have no illness, is often a figment of our needy imagination. Secondly, it's often far more important for some people to be seen to be "together" than to be seen to be needy. This is part of their scripting. Underneath the coping exterior is a scared child who learned very early that if he wanted approval, then he'd better not demand too much. Even more, that if he wanted approval (and to be allowed to stay alive), then he'd better take care of either Mom or Dad. These individuals are afraid (unless they decide to change), of expressing their own needs and take care of others instead. Often the only legitimate way to get the caring they need (but don't want) is to be ill. Usually one of their parents would have modeled that. And I repeat, these are often the people that we think are coping very well because we want them to be coping very well. "If they can't survive this rat race, then how the hell can we?" They, in turn, need to be seen to be in control.

It is important to note the differences between correlating the social circumstances with the illness, and saying the social circumstances "caused" the illness. This latter position is that adopted by many writers on psychological factors in physical disease. They can see that illness and personal dissatisfaction are related, and therefore believe one caused the other. In this they are not unlike their mechanistic fellows who are still at the point of believing that streptococci cause tonsillitis, or excessive alcohol causes gastritis, or lack of exercise and excessive eating causes obesity. Rather, to take the last example, the lack of exercise is a consequence of depression arising in someone who as a child adopted a loveless script. The excess sugar

Finding the Cause

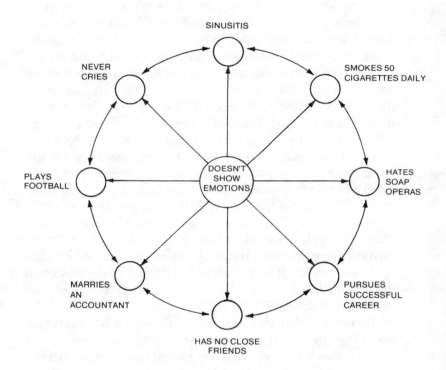

The childhood decision not to show emotion results in the above.

The personal circumstances do not cause each other, for example, smoking does not cause sinusitis, but are interrelated as shown. Changing the original decision will remove the disease and alter those circumstances which were in the service of the original decision and are now disadvantageous.

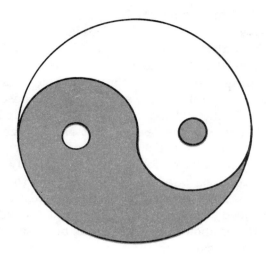

from overeating suppresses the sadness and anger at being unloved, and the obesity renders them unattractive to others and themselves. None of these three features, lack of exercise, overeating and obesity caused the other, rather they were all the result of, and maintained in the service of, the early childhood decision to be loveless.

I have abandoned the linear notion of cause and effect in illness in favor of the cyclical interdependence of mind and body. This is most cogently expressed in the well-known Yin-Yang symbol. Illness, wellness; hot, cold; happiness, unhappiness; light, dark; sanity, insanity; are all a continuum. None is definable.

THE DIET HISTORY

"You are what you eat."
"You eat what you eat because of who you are."

Finding the Cause

"You are—you eat."

Diet has always interested me as a treatment modality, at least since I decided about ten years ago to do something about my own state of health, suffering as I was from a rebellious, adolescent overdose of junk foods. Since then, I have been intrigued with how powerful and effective a tool diet can be when used skillfully. You'll get little sympathy from orthodox medical practitioners for this view, mainly because they regard it as against their interests to have the public self-administer an effective remedy that obviates the need for the practitioner; and secondly, they know nothing about dietetics. It has been said that the average American medical receptionist knows slightly less about diet than the average American doctor, unless the receptionist has a weight problem, in which case the average receptionist knows marginally more than the average doctor.

Contributing to this abysmal lack of knowledge about an essential component of human existence are the drug companies, who give most of the money for medical research and who hate advances in any discipline bar their own, and the conservatism of medical teaching authorities. I once heard the well-known English physician Dr. Burkitt say that if he were given the opportunity to improve the health of the people of the Western industrial nations, he would remove white bread from sale and replace it with wholemeal. Such a small change for such major benefit! But as I have said, the reason why people don't do it is because they want to be unwell, or at least prefer illness to confronting certain of their fears.

When dealing with diet, one is dealing with the whole personality, not just an academic appreciation of those things considered edible and nutritious. A

230

careful diet history will reveal an enormous amount about the psychological and personal circumstances of the client. Certain personalities eat certain diets, and changing the diet can alter the mood of a client substantially.

Someone who is flighty and inconsistent will often be eating fruit in excess and, if he wants to calm down, will do better on brown rice and boiled vegetables. Eating excess quantities of red meat may facilitate aggression and bad temper, a decided advantage if you're a professional football player. Vegetarians, on the other hand, may be so placid that the world treads all over them. The lack of adrenal stimulation from eating only vegetables results in a low level of aggression in an often already placid individual.

Most people, I think, would have some image of the eating and drinking habits of different members of the community. Those images are no doubt stereotypical but sufficient for my purpose here, which is to show that diet, like clothes and cars, is indicative of the personality. The owner of a bar is expected to drink large quantities of alcohol. A writer is expected to be slaving over a typewriter with a coffee in one hand and a cigarette in the other, while businessmen are expected to be seen emerging, bloated from food and alcohol, from better restaurants. Eating habits reflect the social movements of people, such as how often they eat at home or out, and how much money is spent on ingredients. Garbage collectors have always claimed that it's possible to tell the personalities of the inhabitants of a household from their garbage. I'm considering asking clients to bring in a rubbish bin so I can rummage through it and save myself an hour of interrogation!

Eating is one of the last free choices people have. While the foodstuffs themselves are far from free, and finances are clearly limiting, within a range we can choose the food we want to eat without interference. This means that those choices will accurately reflect an individual's wants at that time. In the case of children, compliance and rebellion, acquiescence and anger, are all expressed through food acceptance or refusal. Those patterns have a habit of lasting into adulthood and when people eat a certain way, they are often still rebelling or complying with parents' wishes. It makes things interesting when the doctor attempts to change the diet. Immediately the client is confronted once again by someone telling her what to eat; more often than not, this will precipitate emotional catharsis. It's therefore an exceptionally effective diagnostic tool, comprising both the original diet and the effect on the personality of a change in that diet, as well as the physiological effect of the vitamins and minerals. Orthodox dietetics often lack this psychological perspective, depending as it does on a simple balance of the constituents of foodstuffs—the fats, carbohydrates, proteins, vitamins and minerals.

Diet is of such importance to our health that I intend fuller dissertations on both diets for acute problems, and long-term prudent diet, in Chapter 14— Remedial Dietetics and Prudent Diet.

11

The Psychological Profile

BEYOND STRESS

If I believed all illness to be a consequence of stress, and that an investigation of the client's social circumstances would reveal the source of that stress, then my history taking would be complete. However, I believe instead that people construct circumstances for themselves, which they then react to with stress, that is, they are not being stressed by external events beyond their control, but are stressing themselves. Therefore, I need to expand my investigations to include the first times in their lives they made decisions that resulted in stress. That time is in childhood.

The child, forced by parental pressure to make a decision he is ill equipped to make, responds with stress and makes an adaptation. As an adult he no longer needs parents to keep him alive, so he no longer needs to continue with the adaptation or script decision. Stress is a consequence of the grown-up failing to relieve his own internal little kid from the burden of the early decision. With no protection from the parent and adult parts, the little kid is as stressed in the grown-up as he ever was in the child. As a child his options were limited, but as an adult he can expand these and get the grown-up parts to assume responsibility for his decisions. With the pressure off the little kid, he is no longer worried and can decide to do things differently. This process represents the protection part of successful psychotherapy, that is, the client's grown-up part protecting his own little kid.

All illness is a consequence of stress; not stress arising from an individual's immediate environment but left over from a time in childhood when survival made an adaptation necessary. The current stressful circumstances are acting in the service of the unresolved early childhood conflicts. Until people decide to change, they'll continue to set up stressful events in their lives. This reconfirms their childhood decision and helps them feel safe. Illness may result from this stress and may also provide the discomfort that initiates the individual changing, that is, the physical discomfort eventually exceeds the psychological discomfort which spawned it.

Stress, like illness, is assumed to be beyond the control of the individual. In reality it is self-created, and a synonym for fear. The fear can take many forms, such as fear of not making a deadline, fear of failure at sport, fear of losing the love of a spouse, or fear of not earning enough money to support children. These are all considered to be unavoidably stressful but are really personal reactions to situations, rather than stressful situations themselves. The stress is old fear.

An example of how a stressful early childhood decision will repeat itself later in life, and lead to disease through fear, can be seen from the following: The first born child in a family of eight, particularly if she's only a year or so older than the next child, will often be required to help her mother look after her brothers and sisters. If she were under no pressure to do so she would have no more than a passing interest in the welfare of young infants, and would be too concerned with her own life and needs to respond to theirs. Being too young to take responsibility for herself, she can hardly be expected to care for anyone else. That she does so, and does so very well, indicates the active encouragement of her parents. When she cares for her younger brothers and sisters she's told by her mother, "You're a wonderful girl; I couldn't do without you." The message to the young girl is interpreted as being, "We love you (and will attend to your needs) because you're selfless." She really wants to play, eat, sleep and be cuddled by her parents but finds she gets less approval from them if she does what she wants, than when she cares for her younger siblings. She is stressed by this. She decides to get her parents' attention and love by forgoing her own needs and looking after the others. This stresses her as well but less than having to contend with a mother who is covertly hostile towards her for not helping. Children will make whatever adaptations they feel are necessary to attract the love and support of their parents. This is the innate survival mechanism of human beings.

For the next fifteen years the girl grows up taking care of her brothers' and sisters' needs, her mother's fatigue and her own fears. The caretaking becomes a significant part of her personality. She will often marry a man she can take care of. Provided she doesn't change and doesn't get tired herself, she'll probably be content and healthy. If she does change or get tired, then she's likely to become ill.

Finding the Cause

The following format establishes the early child decisions and how they result in certain personalities suffering from certain diseases. It's variously called a personality profile, psychological profile, psyche profile or script questionnaire.

REGRESSION

Worst Scene

Describe the worst event in your childhood. If you're able to recall several that you would put in that category, then describe the earliest one.
What happens?
Who's there? Mother, father, grandparents, siblings, friends?
What are you thinking? Make up a short sentence to summarize your position.
What are you feeling? (happy, sad, scared, angry or combinations)
What are you deciding to do in the future as a consequence of what has happened?
What is Mother thinking, saying, feeling about you?
What is Father thinking, saying, feeling about you?
If either parent was not present, then put them into your fantasy, and make up what you think they may have said, thought or felt.

Best Scene

Repeat the steps used for the worst scene.

Favorite Fantasy Character
(storybook, television, comic book, cartoon, etc.)

Who is it?

What is special about him/her for you?
What was his/her motto in life?

Life Fantasy

The next step in our inquiry is for you to imagine
that you've been born, that you've lived your life
and that there's a point at which you die.
How old are you when you die in this fantasy?
How do you die?
Where do you die?
Who's at your funeral? List them.
What are they saying, feeling, thinking about you?
Now imagine that on your gravestone is one short
sentence, which summarizes your life.
What is that sentence?

Present Life Heroes/Heroines

Who are they?
What do you like about them?
How are you like the heroes/heroines and how do
you differ from them?

Birth Inquiry

Tell me what you know about your own birth.
Are there any family stories or jokes about your
birth?
How long was the labor?
What type of delivery was it? (natural, induced,
Caesarian section)
Was the birth early, late, on time?
Who was there?
Were you a planned pregnancy?
Did your parents want a boy or a girl?

Who chose your name?
What is your exact name from your birth certificate? (If unsure, obtain a copy.)

Parents

What's your mother like?
What's your father like?
Imagine you've just won a race. What does Mom say? What does Dad say?

Name

Nhoj. That's a word in the Martian language. You have never heard it before.
Pronounce it. What does it mean?
Following are the first letters of the four words in a sentence. Complete the sentence. It need not be grammatically correct.
N........ H........ O........ J........

INTERPRETATION OF THE PERSONALITY PROFILE

Regression—Worst Scene

From his language, it's possible to tell which sensory system the client prefers, auditory, visual or kinesthetic; is he *hearing* what was said, *seeing* how his father looked, or re-experiencing the *movement* that took place. This information can be used at a later date to get access to the client's subconscious, and help in both diagnosis and treatment.

The racket feelings, those frequently expressed feelings that remain from childhood, in fact from the very scenes that the client is now describing, will usually be the first expressed. In other words, the worst scene of childhood will contain elements of a person's life, which were traumatic to him at the time and are still causing him anguish as an adult. Racket feelings will often be used to deny underlying feelings that the client finds more difficult to express. Men, for example, may be angry in order to avoid feeling sad and to avoid crying. Women may cry rather than show that they're angry. The men may develop sinus congestion from not crying and the women may develop high blood pressure from suppressing anger. The worst scene usually brings out the racket feelings. When a client tells you about the bad past, he's really telling you how bad it is for him now. He keeps the scene alive in his memory by frequently recreating it in his life as an adult. The energy for doing exactly the same thing in his life now comes from the fear of changing. Those events in childhood, which "spring to mind" in both the good and bad scenes do so because the factors that generated them are still operational. By inviting clients to talk about past events, they will tell you what is happening in their lives *now*. When they stop operating out of the past they'll drop the memory, or have no energy for recalling it.

Often a decision that the client has made that is continuing to affect his life will be obvious here. The pressure he was under can be assessed from the danger to himself during the worst scene. If he was being physically abused by his drunken father, a decision about his safety would have been more prudent than it might have been in the event of a threat by his mother to suspend his pocket money. In the former case the child decision will be longer lasting and produce greater pathology than in the latter, although the number of times such situations occurred is equally important. Clients often express veiled anger at one parent for not protecting them against the other. The parents' comments in the worst scene will often be the injunctions and the drivers. (See Chapter 2—The Childhood Basis of Disease.)

If the client is asked what he'd now demand for himself if he found himself in that situation again, an assessment of his current awareness and will to change is possible. The woman who was sexually molested by her father and is not prepared to acknowledge her feelings about it is likely to continue suffering from herpes until she admits to herself that she was angry about it and decides to drop it.

Regression—Best Scene

If the scene described takes place away from the family, the likelihood is that there wasn't much joy within the family for that child. Some clients have trouble remembering a good scene at all, in which case they led a very somber childhood and will probably be having little fun in their lives now, or at least will be nervous about it. As soon as they begin to feel happier than they "should," they may give themselves a minor complaint to take the edge off their happiness. Headaches, colds and ringing in the ears are favorites.

The thought of the parents in the best scene will often give clues about the drivers. The support or condemnation of children by their parents when the children are enjoying themselves is at the heart of people deciding whether life is to be enjoyed or to be suffered. It's not difficult to see the role illness has in the latter case. Very often the good scene has some distinctly unpleasant (to my mind) ending to it, for example, "I was down the creek playing doctors and nurses with the boy next door, and it was really exciting. Then my elder sister found us and told Dad." In this person's mind pleasure is quickly followed by reprisal of some kind. Guilt and ensuing genital tract dysfunction is likely.

The best and worst scenes will indicate the sorrows and aspirations, the fears and resentments, the wants and the dreams of the client. They will give an indication of how far the client intends going in therapy. If either the best or the worst scenes involve illness of the client or of others in his family, that is, the reaction of the family, particularly the mother and father, to illness in the client, and the reaction of the client to illness in either parent. In addition, the reaction of parents to other family members who are ill will often shape the attitude of the children to illness in themselves. If not directly causing the illness, these factors will have a bearing on the sufferer deciding to maintain or remove his discomfort.

Favorite Fantasy Character

The appreciation of characteristics in others indicates those things we like and don't like about ourselves. If Peter Pan is the favorite character, the client will often regard not growing up as a good thing to do, since Peter Pan himself did not grow up. This is known as a "don't grow up" injunction and, as mentioned previously, is often the child's reaction to a mother who has had several children, the last of whom she encourages to remain at home. The response of these individuals to illness is usually childlike, wanting intense caring and no responsibility. This means that when they're needy they're likely to make themselves ill.

A knight in shining armor may indicate a rescuer,

whereas a maiden in distress may represent a victim. (A discussion of the Game Triangle is to be found in Chapter 15—Individual Psychotherapy, on pages 295-96.) Rescuers usually look after others until they realize they're unhappy themselves. The good health that they have enjoyed for years, and that has enabled them to be caretakers, is replaced by a significant illness intended to attract love for themselves. However, it rarely works, and resentment is generally the outcome. Victims are nearly always suffering from some complaint, however minor.

Superman was my favorite character as a child. I was very unwilling to see the Superman movies when they came out for fear of spoiling the illusion. I saw myself doing great and selfless deeds, which brought me accolades from my fellows and love from my parents. There was little acclaim of the ordinary in my house. It's not surprising that I'm pioneering a new system of health prevention and treatment while my peers are dispensing drugs and driving Porsches. Self-denial was part of the fantasy. By the smile on my face when this book becomes successful you'll see that I've decided to enjoy my abilities for myself!

The favorite childhood character will give an indication of the script that the person has chosen for himself. The script, like the character, may be a winner, loser, banal or tragic. Illness, being part of the script, will usually have a significant role to play in its fulfillment. People with winner's scripts do not, in my experience, die at thirty with cancer.

Life Fantasy

An adult who fantasizes that he has died at ten when he's already forty has a "don't grow up" injunction. Similarly, one who claims that he lived two-hundred years will not want to grow up either.

Death imagined by violence or suicide suggests a "don't exist" injunction. This person is in danger of having a fatal "accident" or contracting a fatal disease, particularly if he had fantasized an early death. In therapy a contract to stay alive is warranted.

The comments made by family members at the funeral will elicit the failures of the individual as he sees them.

> "What does your father say?"
> "He doesn't bother to come."
> "Put him there and see what he says."
> "I knew this would happen (vehicular accident) he never could get anything together, I'm thankful no one else was killed."

Or in the event of a pneumonia gone wrong:

> "He always was the sickly one. Thank goodness the rest of us have strong lungs."

Notice that in both of these common fantasies the client is fulfilling both a family fear and a family prophesy. His death is condoned by the family. Grieving for him rebalances them.

Imagine a single sentence that would fit your own gravestone. Does it show the love of you by yourself and others? Is it angry and disillusioned? Correlate your answer with your health.

Present Life Heroes/Heroines

These choices generally indicate the personal characteristics that the client believes his parents wanted for him. (Wanted him to have for their own needs is more accurate.) In a person with a "be perfect" driver, they are never achieved and this serves the purpose of constantly reminding him that he falls well short of the standards required of him. Someone who wishes to remain angry at his parents rather than assume full responsibility for himself will make himself as unattractive as possible and then idolize a glamorous personality. Someone who has decided to be as physically incompetent as possible may make a hero of a famous sportsman. This reminds him of how clumsy his father told him he was.

On the other hand, people may achieve the goals they set themselves as embodied in their heroes. If they do this for themselves, and not in the hope of parents loving them better, they'll be able to enjoy their success and will most likely be healthy.

The difference between the client's achievements and those of his hero will give an indication of whether the client is a winner or a loser, the severity of his medical condition and how much therapy may be required.

In general terms, the difference between what the client is and what the client says he wants will indicate the drivers and the injunctions. (See Chapter 2—The Childhood Basis of Disease.)

Birth Questions

"When I was born, Mom reckons she tried to give me away, but nobody would have me." Laughter follows.

"My father said I looked more like a skinned rabbit than a skinned rabbit. He figured I'd run like one when I was older."

"Aunt May said it was the happiest day of her life. All those girls' clothes she'd knitted would finally be used. After four boys she was beginning to despair."

"Dad said Mom would ride over rough ground and hope nature would take its course."

The first and last subjects of these examples may have decided that they were not wanted, may have decided not to live and may have had an "accident" or become seriously ill. It depends on whether the parents adapted to the new baby and came to love him or not. Very often the parents' resentment will remain below the surface, even though the child's needs are met. The second client may fulfill his father's wish for him to be a runner or, if it's more advantageous for him to do so, rebel and become fat and slow. Client number three rejoices in being female, has regular, trouble-free menstruation and no vaginal infections. She can admire her own body in the mirror.

Anxiety surrounding the birth of an infant often predates similar anxiety about raising the child. We have seen before how parental fears will usually be taken up by the child who then becomes unsure of himself. Fear of not being able to survive in the world is perhaps the greatest cause of illness.

The needs of parents to have boys or girls, irrespective of the sex of the child, we have spoken of before. If Mother wanted a girl, Shaunine, and a boy came along, then he may have been called Shaun. If he was expected to take care of Mother's needs for a girl, and was stroked for "feminine traits" and not masculine ones, he's likely to be feminine. This is a "don't be a boy" injunction. Mother is unlikely in these circumstances to physically stroke his genitals, and he in turn is likely to adopt her attitude that there's something unacceptable about them. His penis will be smaller, his testicles smaller, his sperm count lower and his sexual encounters less enjoyable in this event, and his predisposition to sexual diseases, such as non-specific urethritis, gonorrhea, dermatitis and herpes will be greater. Many people have learned that they have been adopted when they applied for a passport and saw their birth certificate for the first time. This may put a new light on their medical history.

Parents

The modeling available to the child will be apparent from his description of his parents. It doesn't matter that his opinion of them is biased, it's his reality we're dealing with. From his description of his parents will come an impression of whether he has fulfilled their aspirations, or whether he has failed them. Constructing imaginary situations and noting parents' reactions to them will confirm the scripting. For example, imagine you've just won a race and your mother is there. What does she say? Or imagine you've failed to graduate. What does your father say?

Name

The word I have used is my name, John, spelled backwards. The client's own name is written backwards and he's invited to pronounce it and then to give it meaning. He's not told that it's his name, although often he'll notice that it is. The object is for him to freely associate with his own name.

When he writes a sentence using the letters of his name spelled backwards to form the first letters of the words in the sentence, the last word will often be his name, for example, when John becomes Nhoj:

Now   Here   OK   John.

This is often revealing, as in Percy:
    You   Cancer   Reveals   End   Percy.
Or, Janet:
    Together   Ever   Now   Attains   Janet.

Percy is likely to have more of a problem than Janet. Some people don't insert their own name as the last in the sentence. What do you make of that? You may recall that when I take the history I am listening on one level and observing on another. I have expressed this previously by saying that the content is often not as important as the way in which it is said. This is certainly true of the psychological profile.

A young man with digestive problems was telling me that he was better than his two older brothers at sports. He then added that he was also better than they were at his studies. As he was looking up at me and asking, "Will you love me, Daddy, now that I've been so good?" and, "Please don't make me prove myself again," his tentativeness was because he knew that however well he performed, his father was unlikely to give him the unconditional love he had craved all these years. He was both proud and unfulfilled by his own success. It had not been effective in getting him what he wanted, and his gut problems both reaffirmed his incompetence and gave him a suitable excuse to stop performing. Even his father knew a sick man when he saw one. All this information was available from a combination of the content and the process of that simple statement.

This completes the psychological history. Much more detail will be offered by the client during therapy, at a rate, which is safe for him. I now have a good idea of the factors that initiated the illness, and the unresolved conflicts that are maintaining it. Whether or not the client makes use of his new awareness (I keep him informed of my mental processes as we proceed) will depend on how much he wishes to risk at this time. I respect his need for safety and am careful to distinguish between what he wants for himself and what I want. This is often difficult for me, as Superman tends to hurry things along.

Allowing rather than forcing the client to change, and providing a safe, caring environment are the essential prerequisites to the next step, the healing process.

12

The Illness Option

The first car Ted owned was a Morris Minor. He bought it nearly ten years ago and it wasn't great then. Now the engine had just about given up and the mechanic who had serviced the car over the years had declared that death was at the most three months away. Ted needed a new car. He drove the Morris down to the local dump, figuring that this way he could save the cost of towing the car when it finally broke down, and with the ceremony due an old friend, pushed the car over the edge of the cliff. He went back home to look for a new car in the newspaper.

Being a student, he found that most cars on offer were well above what he had intended to pay, and even noticed a few Morris Minors like his old one for sale. Not having a car made it very difficult to get about and look for a new vehicle. He began wondering what had possessed him to throw away something that was still of value to him before he was sure that he had something better to replace it with.

Five years later when the gearbox was failing on his Pontiac and the brakes needed repairing, Ted remembered the old Morris. This time he drove the old car around until he had secured a replacement, thanked the Pontiac for its reliable service over the years, and even kept it for old times' sake until he could no longer afford the registration. Then he sold it. Illness looks after us well, though the pain, like a leaking radiator, may inconvenience us at times and make us downright miserable at others. When we decide to get the advantages of illness for ourselves in new ways, we can retain the old way of behaving until we have practiced the new way and are totally familiar with its operation. There's no advantage in throwing it away before an alternative is established, and an appreciation of the role it has played is a good place to begin looking for a replacement. By so doing, we learn what we did last time and decide what we can do next time.

Illness is an option. It may not be perfect, like the old car, but if it saves us from doing things we find more scary or unpleasant, like asking our wife if she loves us, or walking to and from work, then we are benefiting from it. It may be the direct physiological consequence of years of unresolved fear, sadness or anger left over from childhood. It may be the way we choose to stop taking responsibility for ourselves and keep ourselves beneath the umbrella of parental care. The old parent may of course be replaced by a surrogate parent such as a doctor, lover, spouse or our own children. It may be a behavior learned directly from a parent, the media or relatives. "If you feel overworked, it's OK to have asthma." Illness is a way to obtain love, to get out of work. It confirms the world as slightly unhappy or perhaps downright miserable, confirms our belief in fate, or provides a drive for success. There are many other uses of illness. All of them were chosen by us as children without realizing it, in order to make ourselves feel safe in the world. They were valid options, selected at a time when we had few or no alternatives.

Therapy involves simply maintaining the old option or illness while new ones are discovered and practiced. In such a manner, Ted from our story retained his old car until he no longer needed it. Eventually, at a rate that is different for everybody, the old choice of disease is "put out to pasture," returned to only under extreme duress and finally removed when the person is confident he or she no longer need retain it as an option. These are the mechanics of the cure of illness.

Let's look at an example of a young child choosing illness. Baby Peter was only six months old when his mother became pregnant again. By the time he was a year old, he knew that an exciting event was about to take place in the family and that things would be different, but the exact implications for him were unclear. Up to now, he had enjoyed the complete devotion of his mother to the exclusion of almost everything else in her life. It was a position of security he enjoyed immensely.

Soon after the new baby arrived, and despite his father taking time off work to take care of him, Peter realized that the days of his mother's undivided attention were well and truly over. Needless to say, he was distraught at this, being only fifteen months old himself and needing his mother as much as before. To his infant mind, the new baby took mother's valuable caring away from himself and this was a serious, even life-threatening, event.

About this time, he was pushing through a new tooth, and this, coupled with the fact that he was caught with his father in a freak rainstorm, resulted in his developing a fever. Much to his astonishment and delight, his mother, who he feared had almost abandoned him for his baby sister, became suddenly very attentive and stroked him off to sleep. The next time he became unwell a similar thing happened, and the next. Eventually it became obvious to his parents that these fevers were attention-seeking. Before they could take remedial action, Peter had developed another fever so serious that he had a fit. His mother was distraught, blamed herself for not caring enough for the older child and, on this and subsequent occasions, called in her own mother to look after the new baby while she looked after Peter.

The fits were so effective in getting his mother to drop her other commitments and concentrate on him that Peter incorporated them into his pattern of behavior. Tests in the hospital revealed the usual pattern for epilepsy, and the whole family put a tremendous amount of energy into his illness.

Peter, while not causing the initial fever, used this mechanism to be cared for. He learned the behavior and, because of its effectiveness, maintained it. Meditation practices can enable some people to *directly* control body functions (such as temperature), and schizophrenics sometimes have the ability to exert direct control over body processes. Most of us are not in touch with our autonomic functions to such a degree and therefore control our bodies indirectly.

Diagrammatically, Peter's case looks like this:

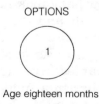

OPTIONS

1

Age eighteen months

The original decision was made under parental influence by a child with little power. That is, to get Mother's attention away from the new baby, the child decides to suffer from epilepsy.

As an adult, the client is able to take care of himself. He marries a nurse from the neurological clinic who supplies his drugs and is up with the latest information on the disease. When their first child is born, neither can understand why this joyous time should be marred by his suffering almost continuous severe epileptic attacks necessitating increased medication and eventual hospitalization.

The fear of not receiving adequate attention precipitates an attack of epilepsy, exactly as it did in childhood. At this stage of his life, he is using only the option he learned in childhood, and as a person who wants to stay alive, this is his best bet. He may or may not be aware of what is happening, but he's afraid to use any of the other options available to him as an adult who no longer needs his parents' approval. That solution worked then, was incorporated into his personality and he became Peter the epileptic. Diagrammatically, this looks like this:

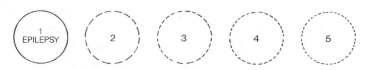

Age twenty-seven years

The epilepsy option is still operational. The other circles represent those alternatives available to him as an adult but which he has chosen to ignore, is unaware of or has considered and rejected. They are all capable of easing his epilepsy but their choice is attended by fear. Some of these alternatives might be:

1. Get a guarantee from his wife that despite the new baby, she'll still have time for him.
2. Ask his wife to reaffirm her love for him.
3. Get a friend who has no child-minding commitments to come over two nights a week and rub his shoulders.
4. Put the child up for adoption.
5. Address himself to his fear about not getting looked after as a child, and look at how he can best get taken care of while he's in the process of deciding to now look after himself.
6. Escalate the epilepsy into the early signs of multiple sclerosis.
7. Drop the epilepsy as being a lousy way to get cared for.
8. None of the above.

There are softer and harder options, and their choice will depend on how life-threatening the child perceived the arrival of the new baby to be. If the mother was very sure that she wanted to have another baby, and the child perceived her obvious pleasure, he may not be seriously threatened by the new arrival. If she were unsure about her ability to take care of yet another child, then the child would rightly fear his needs might not be met. As we have said, this starts him worrying about whether he'll be able to survive this new event and any behavior he stumbles upon at this time, which results in his mother putting more energy into him will be repeated. In this way, the parent or parents condone the child's choice. This, we have seen, is called a "script decision."

The fever which accompanies an earache may be

escalated by the child into a fit if he finds this is effective. The benefit comes from the parents' increased caring for the child, and they have unwittingly validated illness as an option and guaranteed its repetition.

Science is increasingly discovering how physiological reactions, previously considered out of our control, are actually a consequence of the autonomic nervous system reacting to our mental state. Hence, those psychological responses to our environment that are unconscious are continually modifying our physiology and our anatomy. By such a mechanism, the child develops epilepsy. Previously, doctors would have explained the onset of the disease as fate, chance or, more popularly, a virus. Quite specifically the child decides to have the disease and the body accepts the decision, taken as it is in the interest of the survival of both body and mind. Neither can survive without the other.

If our epileptic is very dependent upon his disease for caring, it's unlikely he'll feel safe enough to simply drop the disease overnight. He may decide, however, that he has had enough pills and he may want to begin taking a more active part in the management of his own illness. In such a mood, he may seek a practitioner who elaborates his options and uses techniques to help him experience the feelings he has blocked or suppressed. He is now at the following stage:

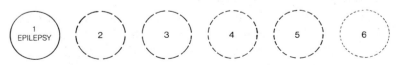

Age thirty years

The illness option is still operational. Peter is aware of options two and three, and beginning to practice them. These will be the options that he finds least threatening. The remaining options, although perhaps leading to a quicker resolution of the illness, are still too alarming for him. For example, he may be willing, in the early stages of therapy, to ask his wife for a back rub, but be afraid to directly discuss the symbiotic nature of their relationship for fear of losing her support. Even later, the couple may want to discuss whether their relationship can survive without the illness. His fear that his wife will feel threatened if she doesn't have a sick husband will often be well grounded. After all, her scripting was that one wasn't a good wife or mother unless one was caring for sick people. If one wasn't a good wife and mother, one was unlovable, and if one's parents didn't love one, they wouldn't keep one alive. Hence, the wife's role in her husband's disease is active and powerful, and of course this is one of the reasons they were attracted to each other and married.

The lightest-shaded option, the one representing total cure of this disease, may never be exercised. It symbolizes what Berne in his book *Games People Play*, Penguin, New York, 1964, called autonomy, and others know as nirvana, satori or existentialism. Not only will it mean that this disease is removed but also that no other serious ones take its place. This option means the dropping of all the old damaging childhood conditioning, retaining the helpful parental messages, accepting yourself, forgiving those against whom you have maintained anger and rejoicing in taking total responsibility for yourself.

If a person has given himself a life-threatening disease (cancer is popular at the moment), and for his own reasons decides to revoke the original decision and survive, he will for speed choose a more drastic option than he might otherwise have done. When the fear of dying or suffering becomes more painful than revoking the original decision, then the lesser of two evils may be a decision to live. Many people who die from an illness do so in a certain state of calm because they are actually fulfilling what they believed their parents required of them. This may or may not be the case, but remember we are talking of adults who fail to free themselves of childhood decisions. The person who chooses to die young has obviously been under some real or imaginary pressure as a child to choose that option and is too afraid to revoke it as an adult. The force of the original decision and the secret harboring of death as an active option mean that most people will not choose the hard survival option if they are suffering from cancer. They are also surrounded by relatives and caretakers who have an active investment in the patient fulfilling the early decision and dying. Most if not all spouses intuitively recognize that their partner is suicidal in one area or another, and this is a major factor in their choice to spend their life with that person. Similarly, the victim's family, having been an integral part of the original decision, will be expecting the patient to die. In certain ways, this restores the balance of their own lives.

When the general consensus is that the patient should die, it takes a lot of courage to choose the hard option of survival. The alternative is to follow the original script decision and die. The lack of fear is seen as serenity and bravery by those around, and I recall as a medical student the aura of excitement when a younger patient died on the ward. It was as though that person had done us all a favor by choosing to die and, as a consequence, improved our chances of surviving. It was similar to the practice of some Eskimos, where old people walk out into the blizzard to die and thereby guarantee the survival of those left. We are not so sophisticated that we don't jostle for survival.

But back to our man with the epilepsy. He has tentatively begun practicing options two and three. This is seen in the diagram as a darkening of the circles as those options are practiced. There are many options, which he may have considered and already rejected, such as having the baby adopted. Whether he continues to remove his disease or not depends on what level of discomfort, or what sort of discomfort, he is prepared to trade off against his fear of becoming completely well. Epilepsy, for example, is an intermittent disease. It is very convenient for short bursts of total disability that require complete care. Between attacks the client is usually completely normal and can get on with following a successful career. It will therefore be chosen by someone who needs temporary, rather than permanent, incapacity, as might be provided by severe arthritis. It's also frightening to watch and difficult to ignore, but is easily concealed when there's no benefit in showing it.

If the arrival of the children in the family means that having epilepsy is no longer convenient, or if the wife refuses to continue to regard his illness as her responsibility, then Peter the epileptic may decide to continue expanding his options and considerably reduce the frequency or the severity of the disease, or even cure himself. Some people come to realize the way they have been using their illness through self-discovery, and decide to remove it. I believe most people who make significant changes to their lives do so without the intervention of professionals. Others make changes by finding strength in God or by surrendering to a guru. Most religions work by using a figurehead to give the devotee parental permission to drop both their pain and their illness. As such, they represent the greatest healing ministry on earth and always have done.

As Peter discovers that he has some control over his epilepsy, he tentatively decides to remove it. He is now at this stage:

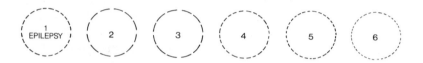

His epilepsy continues to improve and he is well advanced in the practice of the two early options two and three. These, if you recall, were to examine, in conjunction with his wife, the role the epilepsy played in their relationship. As a consequence of them both deciding that Peter has to take responsibility for his condition, they have been less angry with each other these past few months. The bonuses for their relationship will continue as the symbiosis around this disease lessens. In other areas they may well decide to maintain their symbiotic relationship as they both enjoy it. Most importantly, from the illness point of view, as the other options are exercised and practiced, so the epilepsy option is phased out. It is said that the decision to have the epilepsy is old in memory, having been taken all those years ago as a child, but very strong in practice, having been practiced all those years. The newer options on the other hand are weak in practice but strong in memory. The object of the choice of new options is to make them automatic in practice so that eventually being well becomes the usual and expected state of the body. To this end, Peter the epileptic may decide to look at his remaining options.

To be totally free of this disease he may need to become aware of the decision he took to have it in the first place, and be prepared to drop the feelings that he has associated with that decision. For example, he may be still resentful that he was forced to buy his mother's attention by making himself ill. Although he has not realized it, his wife has noticed that he becomes very agitated when his mother begins fussing over some minor complaint in his children. On one occasion she can even recall her husband saying to his mother, "You can cuddle them when they're well you know, Mom!" Aware of it or not, this deep-seated resentment towards his mother about his illness will stand in the way of a cure. Once again, some people deal with this on their own, others require professional help. In the case of Peter's epilepsy he may need to make a conscious decision that he's lovable without his epilepsy, that he no longer needs it to get close to the people he loves, that he can ask for the caring he wants without having to prove he's ill and therefore deserving. He may need to understand the reasons behind his mother's attitude to illness and, having understood the pressures on her, forgive her. Or he may be prepared to do that without any conscious awareness of the factors involved in his parents' psychology. Each individual is entirely different, and their therapy is equally different. Compare this with the treatment of epilepsy by uniform chemical means.

At any point of awareness about his condition, he practices the options that are safe for him at that time.

As the years go on, his subconscious mind will allow into his awareness new and interesting angles on the disease. Diagrammatically, he is at this stage:

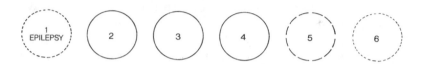

The epilepsy hasn't been entirely removed from his range of options and with many people it never will be. It's no longer a problem, however. Under duress, Peter may choose to return to his disease. In fact, the night his mother died he suffered his first attack of epilepsy in fifteen years. His wife comforted him and was very glad to do it, both really knowing his epilepsy completely for the first time.

Illness is an option. It's a perfectly sensible option arising from the perceived danger of withdrawal of parental support. It enables us to continue to function without the continual fear that our existence is in jeopardy, which is intolerable. It's something we create to allay our greatest fears. It reveals we are prepared to undergo physical discomfort in exchange for psychological security. Simplistic removal of physical symptoms (as in surgery) may unmask the psychological component too suddenly, and precipitate dysfunction. Usually the individual will develop a new disease to take the place of the one so suddenly removed.

An appreciation of the disease—"Thank you, disease, for the way you've looked after me"—is indicative of the self-love necessary for cure. To continue to berate something that is part of you, has developed at your request and has been in some ways an advantage for you is to hang on to the old insecurities and guarantee continued illness. When the advantages in the illness are established, options can be worked out to cater for the needs previously catered for by the disease. When we no longer need the disease, we put it out to pasture.

EPILEPSY—SOME CASE EXAMPLES

Jane was eight and had been suffering from epilepsy for four years. She had a sister, Penelope, who was only a year older than herself. There was another girl who was eighteen months old.

The usual investigations had been performed and an electro-encephalograph (EEG) confirmed the diagnosis. Jane was taking the drugs that are commonly prescribed by doctors to lessen the frequency of the seizures.

When the patient came in to see me she was accompanied by the two other sisters as well as her mother. I was soon to find out why. My first question was "How old are you, Jane?"

"Eight," her sister Penelope answered.

"And where do you live?"

"At 48 Station Way, Pinefield," came Penelope's reply, and for good measure, "telephone 64908773."

"I see, and how much of a problem is the epilepsy for you, Jane?"

"Well, sometimes she has fits and then I watch more carefully when I take her to school in case she has a fit in the middle of the road and gets run over by a car," Penelope answered.

Noting all the time their mother's nods of approval at the answers being supplied by the elder daughter, I'm beginning to see the family dynamics. "Now we're going to play a little game," I propose. This suggestion is taken up with some gusto by Penelope and seeing her sister so enthusiastic, Jane smiles eagerly. "I'm going to ask some questions and I want Jane to answer them, and during this part of the game, Penelope is going to see if she can be very silent, even though she knows the answers to all of the questions."

Of course I'm immediately thwarted in this exercise by the mother, who simply takes over where the brooding Penelope left off, so I eliminate her answering the questions by simply asking her to desist. This leaves Jane squirming at the end of the simplest questions like "What games do you like playing?" and "Have you ever been hit by a car?"

The method this family has worked out to give its members a feeling of being needed and therefore loved, is to clearly demarcate the roles. Penelope, only one year old at the birth of her sister, and furious at this very dangerous intrusion into her life, learns that to get the care she needs, she must appear to love the new baby. Mother encourages her in this, as she fears Penelope's anger and wonders if she'll do the baby some harm. Mother's anxiety about sibling rivalry forces Penelope to take care of Jane to such an extent that the younger girl couldn't even answer for herself. Her epilepsy served the obvious purpose of providing a visible handicap that justified this state of affairs continuing. Jane would play ill and incompetent, Penelope would take care of her, and the mother would feel safe and stroke them both for their respective roles. Therapy in this case was family therapy. There was no point in treating Jane in isolation, because the pressure on her to continue having the illness was so strong. The whole family needed a new range of options whereby they could all feel safe and loved without needing one member to be ill.

We did this over a period of three months, with me frequently congratulating all concerned at a very clever and effective way of sorting out the way they related to each other. Given any set of circumstances, I believe people work out the very best solution for themselves, and at a time when it's safe for them, search for new and more effective options.

The second case of epilepsy that I describe illustrates how orthodox medicine might benefit from taking more time with the history and less time on the routine investigations and then the routine prescription of drugs.

Lisa was sixteen, very pretty I recall, and recently arrived from Canada. She was staying with friends of her family who were worried by her typical grand mal epilepsy, suddenly acquired and at the time of consultation occurring nightly. The woman with whom she was staying was a trained sister at a local hospital, and to confirm the diagnosis, Lisa had a minor fit in the office of the neurologist she was taken to see. She was given the usual barrage of high-powered investigations, which showed the usual result in these cases, that is, nothing abnormal. Nevertheless, to make the case completely typical, she was given a large dose of drugs; I gather that this was because of the frequency of the attacks but, in my view, quite indiscriminately and without proper inquiry at any stage.

Apart from the attack in the neurologist's office, which I put down to sheer anxiety and certainly wouldn't blame her for, the others had all occurred at night. My line of inquiry therefore centered around her thoughts and feelings as she went to bed. She had no recall of any dreams.

She was not easy to coax, being somewhat shy, but eventually volunteered that she was given the responsibility at home of rocking to sleep her younger retarded sister. This was no easy task, but there were six children in the family, and Mother certainly didn't have the time. As long as she could remember, Lisa had rocked the girl to sleep, and if the task was not completed successfully, then the retarded girl would wake in the middle of the night and usually wake the whole family as well, resulting in a major upheaval for which Lisa was held primarily responsible. As a result of the commotion, the retarded girl would often have fits.

As she was drifting off to sleep, Lisa would think of these things and feel guilty that she wasn't at home looking after her sister. In the absence of her family's condemnations she took to punishing herself, and the epilepsy, induced as it was by fear, proved helpful in this regard. Therapy took only one session and involved the girl in fantasizing that the younger sister was being well cared for, which was actually the case, and understanding that she was not her sister's keeper.

I didn't see her again but received a letter from the hospital saying that quite miraculously the attacks had stopped some months previously and hadn't recurred. I looked up my notes and the time corresponded to our treatment session. Much to the neurologist's credit, he took her off the medication.

These cases are intended simply to familiarize the reader with an alternative frame of reference. Rather than attribute illness to external factors, be it virus, weather or pollution of foodstuffs, I interpret them here in terms of the person's early life decisions. The other factors mentioned probably also play a part—they usually do. I believe the early life decisions are the most important and the most ignored of the causes of illness and represent the area of greatest hope in making the great leap forward in the cure of illness.

III

THE TREATMENT
OF ILLNESS

13

Introduction to the Treatment of Illness

I have established a theoretical basis for the belief that people, through unresolved childhood conflicts, make themselves ill. I have demonstrated that careful history-taking and equally careful observation will demonstrate which particular childhood decisions, leading to particular personality traits, are responsible for the illness. Those decisions, we have seen, are reflected in the person's body, his language, his posture and every conceivable major and minor idiosyncrasy, as well as his chosen illness. The personality can thus be used to establish the origins of the illness. Having established how the person makes himself ill, we must now address ourselves to what he can do about it.

The first option available to anyone faced with the prospect of continuing disease is to deny responsibility. We have seen previously how this choice will simply continue the illness. In this instance the client seeks out a practitioner whose interests lie in perpetuating the myth that the illness is beyond the client's control, and both collaborate to provide symptomatic relief without insight. This usually involves drugs or surgery, and guarantees that the illness will remain long after that particular fashionable treatment has been superceded or fallen into frank disrepute. Within twenty years of their introduction, nearly all drugs have been removed from the market, as their cumulative disadvantages begin to overtake their advantages.

The alternative is to seek a practitioner, priest, friend, guru or psychotherapist who can help to expand the options. Ultimately, however, the only satisfactory answer to the client's problems are to be found within himself. It seems that we go through the stage of seeking others' opinions, if only to reject them. We must make the final decision ourselves, and that may be no decision. What follows is one man's subjective opinion about ways to change. Ultimately you will need to reject it.

I work with people in therapy in two ways: individually and in groups. Most people have several individual sessions before they go into a group, and therefore I will start by describing what happens in these sessions.

The immediate history, past history, family history, systems analysis, diet history, physical examination and psychological profile have all been dealt with in great detail. It takes about two hours or two individual sessions to do this. I then engage the person on two levels simultaneously, discussing the role that they have personally played in their own illness, and their diet. While these two areas of treatment may seem incompatible, in practice changing the diet will usually stimulate the emotions. If you are having trouble believing this, I suggest you try a three-day fast before reading further. You'll be feeling quite different in three days' time.

If you're generally racket angry (that is, anger is a common response for you), the change in diet will probably invoke your anger: "As though my headaches aren't enough burden without the additional imposition of this damn diet!"

If you're depressed, then eating may be one of the ways you comfort yourself. Taking away one of your few pleasures may result in you saying, "I don't mind forgoing the white bread but there's no way I can do without my morning coffee."

Or if you're scared, "Where am I getting my vitamins and minerals from on this diet?"

Although under enormous pressure from advertisements to choose one product over another, we still decide what we'll eat. The more pressures we are forced to live under as a consequence of world tensions and our organized society, the greater the attraction of the supermarket. A great variety and availability of foodstuffs, especially those containing sugar, the great anxiety remover, and fat, the soul-warmer, are produced specifically to help us cope with the pace of life. We have become accustomed to this instant, oral gratification and vigorously resist any change in that area of our lives.

When I change client's diets, often substantially, they react. This brings to the surface feelings of which they may be unaware, and injects energy into the healing process. Another way of looking at this phenomenon is from the simple viewpoint that if they want to return to eating recreational foods, then they're motivated to understand the ways in which they are contributing to their illness. The loss of social interaction resulting from the diet (dining out is difficult when you're eating boiled vegetables only) is more painful than an excursion into their own psyche. In this mood they are suggestible.

In the same way as emotions affect the internal organs, physiologically at first and then anatomically, changes on a physical level can affect the way we are feeling. Most people recognize this. Most people are quite prepared to say, "Last week my back was aching and therefore I felt terrible. This week it feels better and therefore I feel great." They are prepared to state that their physical feelings "cause" their emotions. They are less prepared, as a rule, to admit that the way they are feeling "causes" their physical pains. The reason for this lies in the belief we have in this community that emotional feelings are less worthy of sympathy than physical ones. A quantifiable physical pain is good reason to feel terrible. Sadness, on the other hand, is less valid.

The diet changes also affect us physiologically, since the digestive organs are dealing with different foods, and these changes have psychological consequences as well. As I have said, this isn't well recognized but then very few people have practiced remedial dietetics. Unless the physical and the mental, or the physiological and the psychological, are regarded as dynamic or continually interacting, therapy becomes a very one-sided affair, and ineffective. I therefore believe the physical therapies need to take the psychological state into account, and the psychotherapies need to take the physical body into account. When this is done, progress is enhanced. Practiced alone, the physical therapies tend to encourage nonresponsibility and dependence, while the psychotherapies espouse responsibility but encourage transference, and then deal with it poorly. Transference is the phenomenon whereby a client puts Mother's, Father's or both parents' faces onto the therapist or therapists. It's the medium of operation of psychoanalysis. As a consequence of doing this, people don't take ultimate responsibility for themselves but pass it from parents to therapist. Anyone who does this will never get better because to remain under the care of another they need to have a demonstrable illness. In order to guarantee this continued illness, they sabotage the healing procedures of each practitioner they attend. Unfortunately, patients are encouraged in this by most doctors and many psychotherapists who, for their own needs, encourage the transference by counter transference. (The doctor tells, or implies to, the patient that he will take care of him.)

While a change in diet is therefore affecting us by evoking an emotional response, it is simultaneously, by altering the function of the organs, augmenting our reaction. The careful and detailed prescription of diet, taking into account both the physical state and the psychological profile, is called remedial dietetics.

14

Remedial Dietetics and Prudent Diet

The first thing to clarify is the difference between "remedial dietetics" and long-term "prudent diet." The former is a detailed prescription of continually changing diets intended to alter body physiology immediately. Long-term "prudent diet" or the "diet of best chance" is a general dietary prescription that will be of benefit to most people most of the time and, if followed approximately over a long period, will result in general well-being. The diet literature is incredibly diverse because writers do not distinguish between these two forms of dietary practice. The majority of books, and there are thousands of them, are so general as to be completely useless for any particular individual suffering from a set of symptoms. They are written by someone who has seen a narrow range of clients in a particular locality within a narrow time span. In addition, his views are invariably colored by personal preference. A writer who has cured his arthritis by eating boiled vegetables and brown rice will most likely recommend the same diet for others suffering from arthritis. That is absolutely ridiculous. The dietary recommendations end up being generally true, but of no possible use to anyone wanting to change the course of an *acute* illness. To do this an intimate knowledge of the client, ascertained by the previous detailed history-taking, is essential. Clearly this is impossible in a book. I therefore intend discussing a few of the general features of remedial dietetics, and point out that they are applicable to none of you. Then I will list a series of recommendations for long-term prudent diet, which are of value to us all, but over which personal idiosyncrasy must always take precedence.

I've said previously that a person's diet is yet another piece of information with which to piece together the personality profile. Someone eating "take-outs" six nights a week, and eating out of cans the rest of the time, who drinks ten cups of coffee and smokes thirty cigarettes a day is not looking after himself. He needs the instant gratification that his diet provides and will smile perversely when telling you that he always has a hot breakfast: a cigarette and a cup of coffee! He takes pleasure in putting his body to the test, seeing how long it can survive the destructive urges of its master. To force this individual to eat raw vegetables, whole grains and lean, white meats or soy beans would precipitate a crisis. Providing the psychotherapy back-up system is effective, that's precisely the recommendation I may make. Of course I cannot force him to eat anything but neither can he lie to me about those recommendations against which he chooses to rebel. First, there is no point in him not doing what I ask unless he lets me know about it. Second, I follow his excretory functions, sometimes on a daily level, in such detail that I'm able to tell what he's eaten without information from him. You may recall the questions about bowel function (pages 122-4). Conversely, and in my practice more frequently, I am consulted by people with "perfect diets." A perfect balance of cooked and raw foods with an ideal intake of vitamins, proteins, carbohydrates and fats. Fiber intake is sufficient to insure good bowel function. Sugar and salt, along with artificial additives of all descriptions, are kept to an absolute minimum. Much to their horror, I recommend greasy fish and chips washed down with liberal quantities of soft drink of a simply awful nature, followed by chocolates and confectionery, which are difficult to distinguish from pure white sugar! Now to remain on this diet forever would be a disaster, but it can be used very effectively in the short term to energize a client wanting to stop being so perfect (and so unhappy, generally).

These are two examples of prescribing diet to alter a defense system, and are used in conjunction with psychotherapy. Remedial diet is also of great value in altering the course of an acute disease.

A client complaining of a stomach ulcer or of acute irritable bowel syndrome will recover in a few days on a diet of boiled vegetables and boiled rainwater. This will calm the intestine, calm the individual and remove the symptoms far more effectively than antacids or anticholinergic drugs. As the symptoms abate, the diet is altered to keep the intestine exercised at a level that will stimulate recovery, but not embarrass it. The boiled vegetables continue for a time and other foods are added. The program of recovery might look like this:

Boiled mashed carrots
Boiled vegetables
Grilled white meat
White toast, white rice
Stewed fruit (apples and pears)
Yogurt, cottage cheese
Raw vegetables, herbs
Raw fruit
Whole-wheat bread, brown rice
Milk, cheese, butter, margarine
Nuts, Legumes, spices, hot condiments

Increasing gut irritation ↓

As you can see, the symptoms of the case described were such that I began the diet at level two, boiled vegetables. Had the symptoms been very severe, then I would have started with the cooked mashed carrots. The time spent at each level will depend on the rate of recovery, and if the client's symptoms disappear and then return, we may have to go back a step or two. With such a list the client who suffers from these diseases can manage an acute attack, should he decide to have one in the future.

There are other factors in these cases to be taken into account. The client must chew thoroughly, especially when eating carbohydrates, rest before and after eating, not drink with meals, avoid eating fruits with starches as this may lead to intestinal gas, avoid eating anything that is irritating to them personally, eat slowly, in small quantities, and not immediately before retiring.

While the diet is taking effect, the bowels are carefully monitored, as is the urinary output and nature.

Notice how, in the case of irritable bowel syndrome, the remedial diet begins by being *very low* in fiber and gradually increases the fiber content as the bowel is able to handle the additional roughage. Now the treatment of irritable bowel is a *high-fiber* diet, anyone will quite rightly tell you. But there's no point filling an inflamed bowel with fiber when it's not functioning sufficiently well to handle it. It will simply make it worse. This is an example of how long-term prudent diet, that is, increased roughage, may be inappropriate in the short term, when remedial diet is required.

Additionally, other personal characteristics will require the diet to vary between individuals. A client with a stomach ulcer who also has sinusitis will not be allowed dairy products in this acute treatment phase, whereas another with a gluten intolerance will skip the toast in favor of the rice.

At the same time as the diet is taking effect the client is encouraged to look at the advantages of having decided to have this disease at this time. When he's suffering pain and discomfort is a good time to propose a cure for the condition rather than yet another palliative, although proposing self-responsibility at this time will often be met with much hostility. An astute practitioner will intuitively pick his way through this phase, taking care of himself above all else. If the client is happy with the dietary treatment and isn't interested in removing the disease altogether, that's fine with me. I invite him to take responsibility for that decision: "I consciously choose to continue this disease (in a milder form) until such time as I feel safe to remove it."

Health is not an absence of disease, it's a willingness to take responsibility for any disease we choose to give ourselves. I believe that in time self-responsibility implies a continuing improvement in those things over which we have control. It does not imply we have control over everything.

If a client won't accept that responsibility then, after a reasonable period, I stop seeing him. It becomes too great an effort for me to continually dodge the carefully laid traps intended to guarantee that I need him to get better more than he does. In this case I have no leverage and will certainly fail, as well as probably end up feeling bad. I choose not to do that, and may recommend a practitioner whose system of medicine would suit the client's current appreciation of his illness. He may return to me later.

As the immediate problem symptoms abate, so the diet expands, until eventually the client is eating and drinking what he wants. To reach this stage may take between three days, in the case of acute diarrhea, and two years, in the case of extremely severe acne. At the end of the stage of remedial diet, the client is offered the general diet considerations as the best way of avoiding a recurrence, while at the same time avoiding those foods that for him are damaging. In the case of the diarrhea, this might be curry; in the case of the acne, it may be fried foods. In addition the amount of those foods eaten is significant. There is no such thing as a "good' or a "bad" food. Rather are there foods that, for a certain individual, at a certain time and in a certain quantity, are not in his best interest. Writers who propose raw fruit and vegetable diets for all have presumably benefited from such an austere regime themselves. This doesn't mean that such a diet will benefit a single person other than themselves, devised as it was primarily in the service of their own psychological needs. These are unlikely to be the same for any two people on this planet. Such tunnel vision (to which diet experts are particularly prone) demonstrates a woeful lack of understanding of the continually changing face of nature, or the laws of Yin and Yang, that is, that which helps one may harm another.

On a physiological level, there are some generalities that will assist most people in keeping their bodies healthy. At the completion of the remedial diet, which the client has learned and can implement himself if need be, I hand out the following sheet:

GENERAL DIET CONSIDERATIONS

1. Eat a large variety.
2. The least processed foods contain the most nutrients. For example, brown rice contains more vitamins than white rice.
3. Eat the least adulterated foods, that is, those containing as few artificial flavorings, colorings, anti-oxidants, emulsifiers, preservatives, etc., as possible.
4. Fresh foods contain more nutrients, especially vitamins, than stale foods. Grow your own if that it possible.
5. Those foods capable of life, for example, whole grains, will grow if planted; processed ones will not. That which is capable of sustaining itself is more likely to sustain you. Beans (legumes) are another example of such foods.
6. Locally grown foods are generally best. The metabolism of a person living in the tropics is more capable, some would argue, of digesting a mango, than that of someone living on the Mediterranean. Similarly, if apples grow where you live, then you are more likely to be suited to apples than to bananas, which are tropical.
7. Eat seasonal foods, for our bodies are as seasonal as fruits and vegetables and more capable of digesting summer fruits in summer, winter vegetables in winter.
8. Chew thoroughly.

9. Rest before and after eating, as this facilitates digestion by not diverting the blood supply of the stomach to exercising muscles.
10. Avoid drinking large quantities of very cold drinks with meals for cold liquids reduce the blood flow to the stomach, and may remove some of the digestive juices.
11. Observe personal idiosyncrasy—this overrides all the other points. For example, a general diet consideration is that raw vegetables contain more vitamin C than cooked vegetables. However, if you have gastritis, raw vegetables are more irritating than cooked vegetables. An individual condition therefore takes precedence over the general considerations.
12. Socialize with impunity, knowing your body can handle anything you choose to eat in certain quantities.
13. Don't be a fanatic, as mental rigidity tends to negate good nutrition by influencing the absorption and excretion of the bowel.

Under this last recommendation is included all those dietary practices which receive considerable notoriety in the press, and which people seize upon in their ever-willingness to dismiss their own intuitive feelings about what's good for them in favor of a higher authority. They try the new popular diet for a while and generally feel better for a while. Of course, the excitement of doing something new can temporarily relieve all manner of ills. Then the old problems begin creeping back and they realize that they're no better off than they were or, more accurately, no happier. By this time, however, someone equally as clever as the proponent of the first diet has read the political and social mood so accurately that the next diet is on the bookstalls and ready for the gullible. In this, he or she is aided by commercial interests equally receptive to the need of people to be regularly offered panaceas. Until people dismiss all authorities (including myself) as offering no more than broad generalizations of passing benefit, and begin relying on their own internal resources, they will never be healed. In order to maintain that they are in need of help, they cannot, of course, afford to be cured. Until they are ready to trust themselves, their faith in healers serves the purpose of maintaining their own illness.

I am making the point that psychological need is the prime factor in people adopting most popular dietary regimes. Many of these regimes are a return to an eating pattern that was possible in the nineteenth century but totally impractical now. Organic vegetables grown in pure, unfertilized soil, watered with pure water and photosynthe- sizing pure air are just not possible. I believe also that they are not desirable. If our minds and bodies are continually interacting and mutually supportive, then the diet we eat needs to take our current stresses and personalities into account. A nineteenth-century diet will suit only those people who opt out of the twentieth century. To drink soft drink, eat fast foods, dine out at restaurants and eat confectionery is part of the balance of twentieth-century living.

To exceed the limits of a body attempting to adapt to the new chemicals of the twentieth century is to invite physical disease, while a moderate intake of chemicals will insure that the body continues to modify itself to meet modern needs. As with all things, a balance is essential. I presume that if we eat junk foods to a moderate degree, then both our livers and, more particularly, our children's livers will be better able to handle them. The fact that many people use junk foods to moderate their dissatisfaction with life and to suppress their fears is a matter I have discussed elsewhere. I mention it here for balance.

The practice of remedial dietetics is an art, and I have but glossed over it here. The careful prescription for each client, taking into consideration who he is and who he wants to be, is a valuable ally in both assessing and treating the psychological component of his illness. I believe that any treatment schedule is incomplete without an appraisal of the role of both short-term and long-term diet in the causation and maintenance of the disease.

This access provided to feelings by altering the diet is not surprising when the following is considered. The illness we are dealing with is a consequence of a grown-up person refusing to take full responsibility for himself and trying to engage someone as a surrogate parent because of unresolved childhood fears. The greatest fear in childhood is the fear of not staying alive. Food is the prime vehicle whereby a mother passes love and life between herself and her baby. Everybody who has eaten has a food "issue." Food means different things to us all but everyone associates food with being loved and allowed to stay alive. It's logical that altering the diet will have a significant effect.

The beauty of diet in the long-term is the way it dovetails into the psychological notions of self-responsibility, self-love, and continuing self-education and self-care. People leave treatment with a firm connection in their minds between caring for themselves and nourishing themselves with health-promoting food. They have a ready tool whereby they can practice self-care on a daily level, and also be aware of times when they feel ill disposed towards themselves. Nobody can force us to eat anything, and although the diet has been devised by another person, personal wants and individual biases are built into it in such a way that people understand it to be their own. It's still their decision whether to eat healthily or not which provides a safe way for those used to relying on the expertise of others to slowly experiment with their own power. They may rigorously apply the recommendations at first, before risking a few changes and seeing what happens. Eventually, they learn about themselves to such a degree that they are capable of devising their own diet to suit their changing needs.

No therapist sitting in his office, or author at his typewriter, can possibly have the data necessary for a meaningful day-by-day dietary prescription for everyone. Using his guidelines, it becomes up to you. By the client taking responsibility for his own diet, he is in effect parenting himself (parents feed children), and that's the end result of all successful psychotherapy. The lack of transference in this situation is one of the reasons why diet therapy is so unpopular with the vast majority of patients and practitioners. (Transference is the process whereby the client casts the therapist in the role of an all-powerful, all-knowing parent figure who will take care of the client's problems.) I believe that there can be no transference without counter-transference, which is the part the therapist plays in taking on the parent role. I am concerned with transference because, like most of us, I struggle with the fear of being totally responsible for myself. Diet therapy provides a way in which clients can break out of their dependance on therapists. Some therapists don't like that.

In summary, diet as a treatment modality has the following advantages. It provides a physical component to the psychotherapy, thereby balancing the treatment. It involves the client in taking full responsibility for the treatment at an early stage, since he's preparing, administering and taking the prescription. In the long term, diet represents self-nurturing. Clients learn about their reactions to diet in such detail that they equip themselves with skills that they can use in the case of future illness. By so doing, they lessen their dependance on other healers. Diet is the perfect adjunct to psychotherapy as it mobilizes the emotions. Because diet is closely associated with self-worth, self-love and the desire to stay healthy and live, it can be used diagnostically and predictively. Correct, sensible diet is a readily available method for keeping our bodies healthy on a purely physical level.

15

Individual Psychotherapy

My skills as a psychotherapist are derived from my childhood need to survive in a sophisticated, disrupted family. I believe the same to be basically true of all psychotherapists. It seems ironic that these people, who struggled for survival as kids and are now therapists, are deified by clients wanting to attribute wisdom and peace to those who perhaps least have it, certainly who least had it. I do not accept those accolades offered to me by clients wanting me to look after them. Rather do I accept my skills (and sadness at having needed to acquire them) and use them to assist others to assist themselves in their quest for autonomy. I rather suspect that the real test of me having forgiven my parents will be when I cease being a psychotherapist. Until then, this is what I do.

By now the client and I have infinitely detailed the physical ramifications of the client's defense against his fear (that is, his illness) and using the script questionnaire have ascertained what that fear is in general terms. We have some details about how this particular illness specifically allays those fears, for example, how his acne keeps the teenage boy safely away from those women he fears. We have instituted a diet to begin correcting the physical imbalance of the acne, and in so doing have mobilized some feelings. By this time the client is either eager to assess his role in this illness and looking forward to an analysis of it, or rejecting the notion of self-caused illness altogether. Let's look at the former situation, a willing client using a private session. You will recall that I work individually and in groups.

James is twenty-four and has been suffering from severe acne since he was fifteen. He has been to several dermatologists, all of whom have described his case as one of the worst they have seen, and all of whom have administered treatments of dubious safety, with various degrees of desperation and with uniform lack of improvement. James says he's fed up, and that the acne is ruining his social life. He's a computer operator who plays Australian Rules football. His frame is slim and muscular and the rest of the skin on his body is fine and slightly dry. In his face I notice fear, anger and sadness. The anger is most apparent, evident in the thin upper lip and the large jaw muscles. The sadness and fear show in the eyes, the former in the blue discoloration below the eyes and heavy lower lids, the latter in the tension of the surrounding muscles and the intermittent glazing over of the eyes. There's a little dermatitis behind the ears, also indicating fear.

I remembered that James undressed willingly for the physical examination, and that I was surprised to find how large his shoulders were. He was clearly used to carrying a considerable burden. His chest muscles were very powerful and he held them more for protection of his heart than for display, although he obviously derived some pleasure from his own physique. He moved gracefully, holding his buttocks more tightly than most twenty-four-year-old men. They had developed from years of tension and when I touched him on the back they contracted and were rock-hard. His testicles were normal, and his penis, although of normal size, felt and looked enervated. He was more aesthetic than sexual.

The worst scene he described during the personality profile was of him being beaten by his father for something that he didn't do, and then being shamed when he cried. His best scene involved sexual exploration with a girl he knew when he was seven and she was six. This scene, however, was interrupted by his mother, who had obviously waited for something to happen before "discovering" them. He had an erection at the time and once again was shamed by the event. He fantasized dying at seventy-five from "old age," and his wife and two children, all of whom loved him dearly, were at the funeral. His gravestone read "Loved by his family." His favorite character was Batman.

An edited account of James's first treatment session follows.

> "Hi, James, what would you like to do today?"
>
> "Well, I've been thinking about how I might be giving myself acne and I keep coming up with the same thought—all I want to do is get rid of the damn stuff!"
>
> "How's the acne a problem for you in your life right now?"

"Well, take Saturday night. I'm really looking forward to going to dinner with a friend of mine and his girlfriend. There's this woman at the bar who I've secretly admired for months now, and I think she might be interested. What happens? Saturday morning, I wake up with a face full of pimples. I call up my friend and tell him I can't go, but he says 'Don't be such an idiot,' so I go anyway. There's mirrors all over the place, but thank God the lights are low enough so I don't look so bad."

"How are you feeling as you enter the club?"

"Pretty bad. I guess I'm not too confident."

"And what are you saying about yourself?"

"That no one in her right mind would want to know me."

"Go on."

"Well, the girl is there behind the bar, and after about an hour I get up the courage to go and ask her for a drink, hoping to start a conversation. Just as I get to the bar another guy, who I was sure liked her too, sidles up and asks her out next week, just like that! Of course the bastard's got a peaches and cream complexion. I just kept on walking and hoped she didn't think I was going to stop."

"Think carefully. Did you see this guy about to make his move before you made yours?"

"I guess I did, when I think about it. Yes, he'd just begun to move towards the bar when I decided it was now or never."

"Does that timing mean anything to you, James?"

"Do you mean did I deliberately let him

get there first?"

"It sounds like it. What were you thinking when he asked her out?"

"Lucky bastard. It's hopeless, she would've rejected me anyway."

"And what were you feeling?"

"Ashamed and angry."

"Can you remember feeling like that as a little kid?"

"Well . . . yes, in the exercise you gave me to do the other day, you know when I was caught with Suzy next door by my mother."

"Just let yourself remember what that felt like. Close your eyes and be there, with Suzy, and be aware of your mother coming in. Are you able to see or hear her?"

"Yes."

"Good, let's try a little experiment. Will you open your eyes, and move into this chair and act as though you are your mother. Tell little James, in this chair, what you're feeling and thinking."

"You said that I was . . . "

"Be your mother."

"You're a filthy little boy. You should be ashamed of yourself pulling down girls' pants. I'm going to tell your father when he gets home and I hope he gives you a thrashing."

"Come back to this chair and respond to that, James."

"You stupid bitch, leave me alone why don't you."

"What might you be feeling if you weren't angry, James?" I ask, noting the tears welling in his eyes.

"Tell your mother how you're feeling."

"I'm really sorry that you keep picking on me," James sobs out.

"Go back and be Mom, and reply to that, James."

"Well, you're such a naughty boy a lot of the time, you need discipline."

"What's your name, Mom?" I inquire.

"Betty."

"It sounds as though you're pretty angry yourself, Mom."

"Well . . . yes. James's father is away half the time and I have to look after the boy. I even have to do some cleaning to make ends meet."

"Mom, do you know that it's very healthy and normal for children to want to inspect each other's genitals? I reckon you probably did it yourself."

"My brother forced me to touch his, that's what happened."

"It's usually exciting whoever suggests it, Betty, and I'm wondering if that's what you're feeling when you sneak up and catch James doing it. Children really are delightfully sexy."

Betty is silent for a minute. She considers the ramifications of what has been said of her relationship with her brother, her husband and James. Tentatively, she admits a new perspective.

"I suppose there might be something in what you say."

"Are you prepared to tell James that it's OK by you if he plays with Suzy and if she plays with him, Betty?"

Again she hesitates. "Well, he does have a beautiful body and so does she. Son, it's really good that you explore each other, and I love you." Mom begins weeping.

"Switch chairs now and respond to your mother, James," I whisper.

"I love you too, Mom. Dad's away so much and I need you to look after me."

"It's good to cry at times, James."

"Are you aware of deciding to do things differently now?" I inquire, as the crying stops.

"I feel so much lighter!"

"Maybe you no longer feel guilty?"

He nods in realization. "I still think I'm a bit scared, though."

"I'm sure you are. But as an adult there's a grown part of you who's very capable of looking after the little kid in you that's still scared. How might that grown-up part of you make sure that the kid is safe when around women?"

James makes a few suggestions.

I continue. "What benefits do you see from having your acne?"

"Well, it's given me an excuse to feel angry at myself and my mother, and at the same time has kept me away from women. The closer I got to them the more guilty I got and I guess I felt that acne was better than guilt."

"And safer for you to feel angry than sad."

"Yes, I'm beginning to see how I was desperately trying to get Dad to stay at home, but of course not succeeding."

"We can deal with that another time."

"I'd like that."

"Right now I'm wondering if you're prepared to pat yourself on the back for looking after yourself so well in this matter."

In this, the first session, James has moved from a position of believing that he personally had nothing to do with the initiation or the maintenance of his acne ("All I want to do is get rid of the damn thing!") to a part understanding of the role that the disease has played in keeping him safe. Such rapid awareness will not be possible for all of us. Nor is it always necessary, for many people, as I have said, make changes in their lives at a subconscious level, from whence they proceed to work effective and desirable behavioral changes. In a similar manner, the hypnotherapist may evoke a healing response from the client. At this point, James is nowhere near done with the acne. The likelihood is that between now and when I see him next, he'll have used the experience of the first session and the insights he gained to reinterpret the data, strengthen his defenses and end up with the same feelings of insecurity and anger, albeit better defended. Some therapists believe that if the client is not cured in one or two sessions at the most, the therapist lacks skills. I can't help feeling that they're the same therapists who travel a lot, never really following up clients for long enough to see the final result. Instead I believe most people's defenses are well ahead of most therapists' skills, and that the client is totally in control of the rate of personal change.

Not only is the client in control of the speed with which he's prepared to resolve his issues but he also decides whether he will continue in therapy at all. As soon as the therapist wants more for the client than the client wants for himself, therapy is a lost cause. In this situation the therapist has no therapeutic leverage, as the client quickly recognizes the therapist's need to cure him as being greater than his own need to be cured. In response to such an invitation the client will most likely hand responsibility to the therapist and, having accepted it, the therapist is then in an impossible situation. He's likely to become very frustrated from the effort that he's putting into curing this person with no results or, more commonly, results just encouraging enough to keep the game going. The client plays victim and the therapist plays rescuer. Many doctors, health professionals and therapists are like this. They may have developed skills to hide their rescuing, but the client's little kid will recognize it easily.

The positions of victim, rescuer and persecutor are interrelated, as shown by S. Karpman, in "Fairytale and Script Drama Analysis"" in the *Transactional Analysis Bulletin*, 7, no. 26, April 1958, in the diagram of the Drama Triangle or Game Triangle:

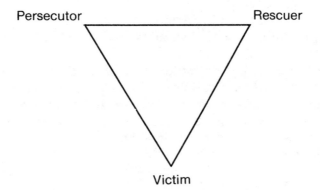

As the game, that the doctor and the patient are playing evolves, they change positions within the triangle. The following is a typical example.

> "I'm feeling very low, Doctor. My sinusitis is terrible. It would have to develop just as I was to go on vacation." (Victim)

"What rotten luck. It must be awful, I'll see if I can help. Take these pills three times a day for five days. That should work." (Rescuer)

"Not more pills. Every time I come here you fill me up with pills. I think it's time I consulted the naturopath down the road." (Persecutor)

"I'm sorry, but that's all I have to offer." (Victim), or

"I told you if you insisted on continuing to smoke you'd pay the price. Stop smoking or have sinusitis. It's that simple." (Persecutor)

Both parties end up feeling uncomfortable because they are involved in a game. In this context a game refers to a series of transactions that end in both parties experiencing racket feelings.

With James I am careful to emphasize the following points. His current state of health, including both his psychological state and his physical condition, is the very best that he could do for himself up until this point in his life. Similarly, I believe he will continue to care for himself as best he can. If it had been safe for him to be unafraid of men and have no acne, then I assume he would have done that.

It was obviously less painful for him to have the acne than to confront some of his fears. Those fears concern his mother's anger at his sexuality, and his father's absence. Most clients take a long time to accept this notion. I know I did. If everything we did looked after ourselves best (given limited options and even less power), then everything we have done and will do is OK. To accept this is to believe that we are OK. If we believe that we are OK now, as we are, then we don't have to change anything. That is unattractive to us for the following reason.

When we were children, we desperately sought our parents' approval, and this meant adapting in certain ways. Much has been made of this elsewhere. If we now make a declaration that we are OK as we are, then we no longer need to adapt. As kids we did need to adapt or suffer the consequences (death, we fantasized), but as adults we no longer need to. However, if we stop paying attention to what Mom and Dad want, either the real Mom and Dad or, more commonly, the parents in our head, then we still believe we risk losing their love. If they stop loving us then who will love us? We therefore cling to the need to be not OK and therefore the need to change, in order to keep our parents loving us (even though they may be dead). And of course it doesn't matter how much we suffer, or how much we change, the love we are seeking, that unconditional love of perfect parents, will never be forthcoming because it is a myth. We create it because we want to be cared for perfectly, we are afraid to be responsible, we are afraid to love ourselves and we are afraid to be alone.

If we accept that we are perfect as we are, and stop making ourselves not OK, we'll need to drop the notion that if we were just that little bit better, Mom and Dad would give us the love we crave. To drop the need to change is therefore to drop the hope of turning back the clock and undoing history. As we become adults we replace our real parents with surrogates such as spouses, the football coach, Jesus Christ, Buddha, the president, Karl Marx, the guru and even our own children. We create problems within ourselves as offerings to these surrogates, hoping that they will see our pain and come to our rescue. We cannot afford to be well.

As I have said, this is often a bitter realization, and people need varying amounts of time to adjust to it. In the meantime they undergo therapy or continually manipulate their circumstances to protect themselves from facing their own aloneness. James will be introduced to these ideas slowly and gently. They will not be forgotten through the hurly-burly and excitement of change therapy. Nor will they be accusingly thrust at him, for he will accept them only when he feels safe to do so, and if he's like the rest of us, his temptation will be to never accept them. Meanwhile his therapy continues.

Therapy has two major components, and therapists tend to broadly orientate themselves into two camps, the "thinkers" and the "feelers." Thinking therapies include psychoanalysis and its modern-day offshoot, Transactional Analysis, while feeling therapies include Gestalt, Radix, Bioenergetics, Primal Therapy, Rolfing and other breath and bodywork therapies. Most therapists tend to use a combination of both feeling and thinking. Hypnotherapy may include both. Those therapists who were brought up to think and not to feel will generally be expert thinkers and poor feelers, while those who decided under parental pressure to express their emotions and not to think about it a great deal will be attracted to the physical therapies. If they are strongly in favor of one and reject the other, you can be sure they are merely repeating their childhood circumstances or rebelling against their parents. That will suit some clients and not others.

James will firstly be encouraged to understand his need for his acne, because I'm more comfortable with thinking than with expressing emotions. He will, however, be given ample opportunity to express the rage and sadness that he feels towards his parents. Emotional catharsis, the outpouring of feelings stored up from childhood, can be very powerful and often frightening to watch. There's no point in James confronting his real parents with the "injustices" of his childhood. It's not their problem. Therapy offers the opportunity to do it. Instead, James is invited to punch or kick a bean bag, or beat it with a tennis racket or a soft baton. I make sure that he doesn't hurt himself, for that would merely confirm his childhood belief that to be angry is dangerous. Equally important is that he doesn't hurt me or anyone else. All the necessary safeguards are taken before he does his anger "work-out." Initially he will be most comfortable expressing his racket feelings, and as he tends to swallow his anger, he will be invited to express it openly and directly. If he has no difficulty in yelling at others, and does so excessively, I will ascertain those feelings that he is covering by being angry all the time. Much anger, apparently expressed in response to an immediate stimulus, is in fact old anger left over from previous incidents. He may be feeling sad beneath his covering anger and, in that event, I will know his therapy is progressing well when he cries in front of me, or he reports crying. In theory, if the old emotions can be mobilized, then they will be done with and the person will re-establish emotional balance. In practice this will not happen unless the bottom level of feeling is unearthed, and that, I believe, is always fear. When fear is dealt with, that is, the client has come to trust himself to keep himself alive and to love himself and get himself loved, he will no longer need the racket feelings and he will drop them. They have served him well, effectively preventing his fear from surfacing. The physical ramifications of these racket feelings, those maladies whose role it was to maintain the old feeling states, will similarly no longer be needed. When James no longer needs to be angry (towards himself and his parents) he will no longer need the acne at which to be angry.

The racket anger moves freely around the circle and draws in outside issues as well, for example, anger at lovers, workmates, or the government. It may be primarily in any one of those three positions at any time and be available to the therapist in that position or indirectly through the other two. The client will regularly move it about in order to thwart a therapist's efforts to contact the underlying fear.

Anger Cycle
Racket anger (shaded area)

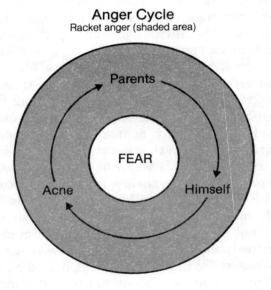

Since therapy continues over a considerable period of time (on average about six months), the reader will appreciate the difficulty in describing the overall process. To report each phase the client goes through in reaching a level of operating that is satisfactory to him, and to fairly describe the therapy of those phases, would mean transcribing the tapes of the sessions. Each client's therapy would occupy a large volume, since no two are alike. Verbatim reporting would show the ebb and flow of progress, for in between the "ah ha" advances, those exclamatory leaps forward in awareness, is the terror of doing things differently as a consequence of new awarenesss, and the tendency to return to old safe ways of behaving. James, our man with acne, may find that mild acne returns at those times when he's most apprehensive. He will learn to use this as a sign to take things easy and to look after himself.

People will always make changes at their own pace, even though the therapist may want them to go quicker. I've had trouble coming to terms with this. When a client starts in therapy, I'm able to detect his basic blocks within the first session or two, and have some vision of what he could achieve for himself. What I really mean is that I can see how dramatic a difference I could make to this man, and how good I would feel to see him leave therapy with his cancer cured. Now what I want for him may have little to do with what he wants for himself, and if I fail to detect my investment in his early recovery, I'm going to be very frustrated indeed. When the therapist is going too fast, the client will thwart the therapist's aspirations every time, even though he will seduce him into believing that they both have similar goals. Subconsciously, the client is sabotaging the therapist's every move. This leads to the often-heard cry among doctors, helping professionals and therapists: "He didn't want to get well." Of course the client wanted to get well, but not in the same direction or at the same speed as the therapist wanted him to. Some clients need to test the water at every step, and that's why for them therapy is a drawn-out affair. It is also why, if the therapist can resist the temptation to push too hard, therapy is so effective. Clients appreciate time to practice new thoughts, feelings, and behaviors before undertaking further change. People don't get better in straight lines. They take two steps forward and one step back, two forward and one back. That is the way the biological feedback systems, which regulate our bodies, work.

Diagrammatically the progress of therapy is like this:

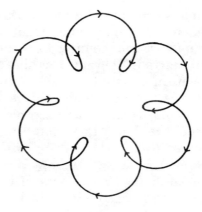

But you end up in the same place you began! What's the good of that? I assume that the place you began, before the adaptations were made necessary and the illness started, was a good place. The illness cycle has been just part of the external meanderings made in an effort to understand who we are and to accept our aloneness. There's no fixed time that we need to have illness, be in therapy or continue searching. We are searching for something that we misplaced, rather than lost.

16

Group Therapy

A lone guitar rises above the sounds of the room, struggling to be heard. The noise settles, the tempo and the timbre of the instrument become sure, obeying every nuance of the master's call. The percussion enters, slowly at first, then gaining in empathy, an accompaniment on a sometimes hazardous journey.

Aware of its fellow traveler, the guitar courses up and down the scales and performs arpeggios with an added confidence. Sometimes in lead, and sometimes in answer, it will engage its fellow, and together they create a new dimension. Their call for others is answered by the bass, a low, rhythmic reply from long ago, before the course was sure, before the celebration began, a reminder of their roots. A violin is the last member of this ensemble. The players' momentum is carved from individual experience, honed by immediate needs to give expression through their instruments, and the need to take part, to share their dreams. The melody becomes clear, the variations and leads are taken and given in nods and smiles as the momentum gathers. Together they see an opening, a way to the unfinished part of their symphony. They combine in harmony against the discord of failure. The audience wills them on. We can feel the dangers, smell the excitement, see the goal. They are in the tunnel, they are racing for the light. The beat reaches for the fury of the occasion, the violin is on the edge of freedom, the guitar hurtles into the void. They explode into sunlight, rejoicing in the singleness of their purpose, in the oneness of its expression. They have made the peak. The breathing becomes easier, the faces peaceful. As the music winds down the audience erupts into a spontaneous acknowledgement of the pain, the risk, the journey, the power and the victory. For a while we are in triumph together. In a few moments we resurface alone.

Group therapy can be very exciting. I enjoy it because of the increased dimensions of people, whose only common ground may be a struggle for love, interacting in a way that shows you rather than tells you how they are feeling and thinking. Individual sessions, although no less penetrating in their analysis, and no less effective in their treatment of an individual, lack the fellow-traveler spirit. Since clients leave the office or the group room and return to a world occupied by others, groups preempt reactions to or by the outside world, by providing a microcosm of that world. This is valuable for clients wanting to practice new behaviors in a safe environment. Every group member, including the therapist, will react to everything said or done by any group member. It's impossible not to react. No reaction is reacting by doing nothing.

Clients are invited to respond on a gut level to the proceedings around them. Those who appear to not be reacting may have suppressed feeling to a level at which they are apparently unaffected by external happenings, or are frozen by fear. Either way it's obvious in their faces, and can be used by both the clients and the therapist in resolving the client's problems. Members will clearly be affected by the issues being worked on by others, and will show it and tell you about it. This level of interaction is not possible in individual sessions. Take the following example.

Bill, who has severe asthma, had been talking to his mother in a chair for some months, on and off. He was still very angry with her and blamed her for his asthma. He was also secretly angry with his wife but wasn't ready to admit it, as he believed that to be angry with another was tantamount to saying you didn't love her. Until Bill was prepared to confront his anger towards his mother as being the way he remained dependent on her, face his anger towards his wife and drop both angers, I couldn't see his asthma going. I resolved to make him uncomfortable.

"Your wife is obviously a real bitch," I told him.

"How the hell would you know, you don't even know her!"

"She married you, didn't she? I'll bet she's like your mother who kicked you around all day."

"What a terrible thing to say," a voice came from across the room, more in righteousness than in anger. "You just don't say those things about people."

"Who in your life is a real bitch, Deborah?" I inquire.

"Nobody, I wouldn't say that about anybody!"

"If you would say it about somebody, who might that be?"

305

"My mother makes me so mad at times."

"Will you see your mother, there, in front of you, and tell her you're mad with her, but you won't call her a bitch?"

"Mom, sometimes you . . . " Deborah begins crying.

"It's OK to be angry with loved ones," I tell her gently, since I'm dealing here with a young child who wasn't permitted to express her anger directly.

"The people we get mad with are often those we love most. Women are taught to cry instead of being mad. When you're ready you might tell your mother that you love her *and* you're angry with her. Meanwhile you're really looking after yourself by not letting yourself get mad . . . Bill, how are you?"

"I'm not sure, I'll think about it."

"Take your time."

From the rest of the group's interest in these proceedings, I know people are in the process of internalizing what has happened.

"What's happening to everybody?"

"If my husband fusses over me once more I'll scream," says Judith Miller, who's almost confined to a wheelchair with arthritis. "He means well, but he makes me so darn angry at times."

"My boss is a real pig," says Stephen, "an arrogant bastard who shoves me around and gets a real thrill from it. I'm tempted to tell him to get stuffed."

"Then what would happen?"

"I'd get sacked."

"Do you want this job?"

"Sure. Right now I can't afford to lose it."

"Then congratulate yourself on keeping cool. How could you keep the job and feel good about it at the same time?

"I don't know."

"Think about it this week, and report back when you come up with something."

"Yes, I will."

By confronting one group member, other transactions yielded valuable information and started others on the way to a resolution of their own problems. Deborah, who's a social worker and rescues her helpless charges as she attempted to rescue Bill in the group, will benefit from getting in touch with her anger. Everybody who rescues is angry at having to do it. When they realize that they no longer have to heal the world as they were encouraged to do in childhood, at a time when they were least capable of doing it, and that in fact they are far more effective if they let other people take care of themselves, they are much happier.

None of the above would have transpired in an individual session. It's generally scary for people to take part in groups, as they feel exposed and vulnerable. Individual sessions are safer for most, as in this situation they need only contend with the therapist, and they have been conning doctors for years. There's no big deal. The group is another matter and is therefore threatening. I do not deny that if people want to move from where they are, they have to risk. I emphasize that groups are great fun, and that a real sense of communion develops in a short space of time. Ultimately, I believe it's very important for people to be able to gradually expose themselves to others. There's something much less effective about telling a client that she's worthwhile, despite being sexually molested by an uncle, when it's treated as a big secret between her and the therapist, similar to the secret maintained between the client and her uncle all those years. In a group it becomes obvious by the failure of the other members to reject the client, and their well-wishes and strokes for having had the guts to tell them, that the matter rapidly defuses. The added dimension of hearing other people, to whom exactly the same thing has happened, tell their stories, further removes the shame, guilt and, even more importantly, the anger remaining towards the perpetrator of the alleged crime. Sure it was sad that the little girl had to have sex to feel loved, sure she can be angry that her uncle needed her to feel guilty to remain undetected, sure she can scream at her mother for knowing it was happening and doing nothing about it. All of that's fair enough. Also true is the fact that not forgiving her uncle will end up in depression and martyrdom. I will not condone the act, nor will I rescue the victim. Unable to tell people of this childhood secret, many people wishing to maintain the energy of the affair will make themselves seriously ill, and carry on bravely. As I've mentioned previously, arthritis serves a martyr well, although in the case above a sexual disease would be more likely. Both will go when the victim drops the need to be unresponsible for her life.

The mention of group therapy often meets with a strong reaction, mostly anger and fear. It's not surprising when you consider that people have been harboring their greatest fears for as long as they've been alive, and have become very proficient at it. The thought of becoming less defended is naturally anxiety-provoking. They will usually mention someone they know who has done "groups," and who has "never been the same since." Some people will attend groups for exactly the same reasons that they've been attending doctors for many years, in the hope of either getting someone else to take responsibility for them, or to blame the incompetence of the practitioner for continuing illness, when in fact they are simply not ready to resolve their problems. When competent group leaders refuse to take responsibility for clients, this reaction may be the client's way of maintaining their dependence. To admit that the expertise of the practitioner is less important than our will to be healthy is to take full responsibility for ourselves.

Physical closeness is encouraged in groups, and people often establish an intimacy that they have previously denied themselves. Getting close to other people, both emotionally (trust) and physically, is very frightening to many people, and this is another reason why group therapy is criticized by those not wanting to risk. I remember a woman who had had a debilitating illness for many years saying to me in a group that she would do "anything to be free of her pain." I replied that she didn't need to do anything drastic, all she needed was to get herself cuddled by any member of the group. She refused.

People are also encouraged to take responsibility for their sexuality, which means that they decide whether they want to become sexually active, or whether they want to suppress their sexuality in favor of a personal contract or perhaps a religious belief. Those who want to practice being sexy in the group can do so. Allowance is made for the prevailing community attitudes to sexuality. Nevertheless, sexual innuendo is a favorite way of dismissing group therapy and unfortunately is yet another excuse for people not changing. Unfortunate, because people need no excuse for looking after themselves. If they aren't ready to accept responsibility for themselves and their diseases, that must be what is best for them. If they can get somebody to look after them, well and good. If they want to do something different later on, they can.

I believe that group therapy has the following advantages over individual sessions in the treatment of illness. First, it's novel. The assessment of illness using psychological methods, including voice, facial and muscular diagnosis, is different enough, but using group therapy to cure people of physical illnesses without drugs is really exciting. When clients are faced with a serious illness and an exhausted orthodoxy, the thought of doing something different, however scary, is attractive. A group of people who gather to forge major changes in their lives, such as healing themselves of serious illness, generates considerable enthusiasm. This contrasts with the lethargy induced by the resignation of doctors towards diseases they regard as incurable. Needless to say, this group energy helps to cure.

Secondly, group therapy is a social event. Clients may have an intimate relationship with their doctors that they both enjoy immensely, but with the great spectrum of personalities present in a group, the atmosphere is even more expectant. Not unlike a good party, groups are used by most people to establish long-term friends. Groups afford one of the few opportunities to know a very great deal about another person before establishing a friendship.

Groups are great fun. I use humor a lot in treatment and a responsive gathering of people is very beneficial in taking the drama out of serious illness. Hanging on to the tragedy of illness is made more difficult when neither the therapist nor the group is enticed into feeling depressed about a disease that someone has chosen to give himself. People usually drop being a martyr very quickly when it fails to have the desired effect. I have found it much more difficult to keep clear of rescuing such individuals in private sessions as they are generally very skilled at getting others to sympathize with them, and will exploit my need to help them, if they can. As I was raised to care for my mother, I am on dangerous ground here.

Group interaction, I have mentioned before, is one of the major components of group therapy. When one woman in the group looks jealous because I'm cuddling another, or the one I'm cuddling shoots a guilty sideways glance at my female co-therapist, then I'm dealing with a couple of little kids responding much as they did in childhood. Both jealousy and guilt will be reflected in their physical health.

By monitoring the reaction of other group members, the therapist is better able to gauge the reality, reason, frivolity or truthfulness of what's being said. I can be sure that if a woman is describing herself being raped, and the group is uninterested, restless or, in an extreme case, yawning, then the story has an element of self-aggrandizement or insincerity. If, on the other hand, the group is listening intensely, they have subconsciously registered that this is an important issue and behave accordingly. In the first case the game of "Ain't it awful" may be pointed out to the client in such a way that she understands that she may do things differently while being supported for having cared for herself. The game was a very necessary defense. In the second example, the woman may be invited to dialogue with her rapist, express her feelings of outrage, forgive him, work out how not to let it happen again, stop feeling guilty and as a consequence stop her dysmenorrhea (painful periods). This will probably take some time. If she's been allowing her feelings to surface, however, she may cure herself overnight.

I may put my arm around a client's shoulder in an individual session, in fact I do so quite frequently, but a group offers a safer environment for physical stroking to be practiced. It also provides information on the fears people have of being touched. Men with a fear of women will get their shoulders rubbed by other men. A woman who is angry with men may snap a refusal at a man who has asked that she rub his shoulders. In turn, a man who likes to be yelled at by angry women will ask such a woman. The sagas of childhood adaptations are played out before the therapist, for him, the rest of the group and the client to see.

In order for therapeutic interventions to work, and for the clients to feel safe to change, it's necessary to establish a caring environment. The tone of voice, the body postures, the honesty of the therapist in pointing out his own areas of difficulty, all play significant roles in this. No acting or conning of clients is possible. Since the client will interpret anything the therapist says to him in terms of his own experience and needs, there's no point in trying to appear what you are not. The greatest factor in any transaction, the need of the client, is thankfully totally beyond the control of the therapist.

Were that not the case, a situation would exist in which the therapist was in control of the client's destiny. That's not possible. My concern for the pain of another involves using my skills to facilitate him achieving what he wants for himself, and in relating to him as an individual who has done in the circumstances the very best he could do.

Cure is the hallmark of group therapy. People actually cure themselves and it's obvious to all present when that happens. To watch a person become happier during the course of group therapy is a very rewarding experience. The whole body changes. The face becomes open and softer. The eyes are untroubled, the voice becomes powerful and well modulated, there's a full range of emotional expressions, there's a willing exchange of physical strokes and compliments are given and received joyfully. The symptoms of the disease gradually abate and eventually disappear, or disappear between one group and the next. To watch this happen is enormously encouraging, or frightening, depending on whether the other clients want to cure themselves or not. Either way it's very effective in mobilizing their energy to accept or resist the invitation.

17

Summary of the
Cause and Cure of Illness

The unborn infant monitors and responds to maternal anxiety. The adaptation begins. The trauma of the birth process confirms the world as potentially dangerous.

Basic needs, which are unmet or met unsatisfactorily, and which the infant is powerless to meet himself, confirm the need to adapt to survive. The child decides that some of his own needs must be modified to meet the requirements of his caretaker. This guarantees continuing care. Some of those decisions lead to illness. Physical and psychological pain develop. The client seeks relief. Drugs or symptomatic treatments modify, or temporarily relieve, the discomfort. The disease process continues. The client becomes disillusioned with the treatment. A level of discomfort is reached at which the fear of the original adaptation is exceeded, that is, it becomes more painful to have the illness than to look at what needs to happen to remove it. The client seeks a healer. He is introduced to the notion of self-cause and self-cure. The client begins to accept responsibility for the illness. He becomes aware of the basis of the illness. His new-found awareness leads him, with the help of his therapist, to expand on those options to which he had previously restricted himself. He decides to do things differently. He retains the old ways until he is familiar with the practice of the new options. The needs that resulted in the illness are satisfied in other ways, and he no longer has any need for the illness. He removes the illness.

18

Perspectives on Psychotherapy— The Transitional Stage

A declaration of cure warrants careful examination. We are all extremely wily when it comes to doing things that make us feel safe. So great is our need to feel comfortable that we develop a very complex system of defenses which are mostly unknown to ourselves, let alone to an outsider such as a therapist. We suppress our fears, our knowledge of them, and knowledge of our defenses of the fears. We are unwilling to admit certain behavior as being defensive, because it's unsafe for us to do so. We are hardly going to inform a therapist of these matters. However, by observing the outward signs of the internal processes, an astute therapist can get a good idea of what the client is thinking, although never a complete picture. Therapy is similarly incomplete, and any therapist believing he can predict what a client will do in the future is deluding himself.

When I say that the client has decided to remove the illness, I mean for whatever reasons. Those reasons may be to please the group leader, the group, the client's wife, his boss or his children. He may have re-adapted in order to remove the symptoms but still be complying with or rebelling against parents or parent figures. If the parent figure is the therapist, which is very common, then transference hasn't been resolved and future problems may arise. Disinterest on the part of the therapist may precipitate a new wave of fears in the client about who will care for him now. Having removed the original illness to please the therapist, he may now have an acute need for something to take its place. Asthma takes over where migraine left off. There may, however, be no reason to doubt the reduced support of the substitute parent. Many people stay very well under the umbrella of Jesus Christ, Buddha or Allah. These days Muktananda, Bhagwan Shree Rajneesh, Swami Prabupada, Gurdjieff, Mahikari or Eckankar play the same role for a generation needing to rebel against parental values but with the same need to be cared for. People who stay happy and well in religious or other organizations have clearly found something which suits them.

When a part of our future happiness depends on the good offices of another, however well meaning and well tried, we're in the position of children. Now Jesus said, "Else ye turn and become as little children, ye shall not enter the kingdom of heaven." Maybe he intended that we put ourselves under the care and guidance of a benefactor, in his case the church, or at least his teachings. As long as we remain true to his word, then we'll be happy and safe. I prefer to believe instead, however, that as long as we remain accountable to another for our actions, and in return receive guidance and protection, either real or imagined, we are limiting ourselves. Certainly we can take into account anything other people say in an attempt to work

out what's safest for us, but to slavishly follow another's advice on how to lead my life doesn't appeal to
me. It may be necessary, however, to do that for a
while. Surrendering to another human being, or a
deity, may be a necessary step towards taking full
responsibility for ourselves. Eventually we realize that
our godhead has not the answers for us that we hoped
he had, and we become our own gods. This may involve the anguish of accepting our aloneness.

In psychotherapy a similar process may occur.
Clients go into psychotherapy hoping to find someone
with the answers for them, someone who'll do better
than their original parents. This new parent will
teach them new skills with which to protect themselves against the world. Very often this is exactly
what happens in therapy. The client comes out better
defended than when he went in, albeit very much better at hiding his fears. In this case he would appear to
have achieved nothing. However, if he realizes that
he's no happier with his new skills, and it may take
some time (it took me three years), he can use the experience to begin to really achieve autonomy. In so
doing he will need to reject the therapy as being no
more than an incomplete theory emanating from the
needs of a fellow sufferer (the therapist) and begin
trusting himself. Most people appear to need to go
through the process of hope, disillusion and then rejec-
tion of the therapy.

As I see it, we're left with a choice to make. That
choice is to remain under the umbrella of another's
wisdom and love or to be our own ultimate master. As
our own guide we can allow the grown-up part of us to
choose another person or persons to help us look after
the little kid in us. The decision to be our own final
authority doesn't imply being lonely. We can surround

ourselves with whom we choose. It does not mean accepting that we're alone in the sense that we cannot
rely on anyone else or any guru to look after us. In a
similar manner, we are unable to ever get inside the
head of anybody else to feel as they do. Such self-
responsibility means accepting that from time to time
we may choose to be unwell.

Some people to whom the notion of being their own
ultimate guardian appeals will be those people who
have experienced inadequate caring as children. They
don't trust others anyway, so are not excited by the
idea of placing themselves in the hands of another.
They do not believe that anybody else can know their
needs or, if they do, will care for them as they want.
They have no experience of this as a child. Their belief
that "I'm responsible for myself" comes from both
their anger and their fear that "no one else will care
for me properly." That's not autonomy, for their belief
is motivated by fear. In a treatment sense they would
be offered the opportunity to place themselves in
another's care, so that they may resolve the fear. When
they trust others to do their best to look after them,
they will believe that they are worth looking after.
They are now in the "I'm OK—you're OK" position, in
which they may choose self-responsibility.

Conversely, others are attracted to the idea of always having an authority to whom they can turn for
guidance. They may in many aspects of their lives be
self-fulfilled, be successful and responsible members of
the community who choose to worship a god, maintain
a guru or stay in psychotherapy forever, sometimes as
a client but more often as a therapist. They have a
sense of great warmth and comfort from believing in
a benevolent god. Without such a belief they feel
scared. Many people adopt religion at stressful times

in their lives and drop it when things get better. They will usually keep their beliefs at the back of their minds and call upon them when needed. I have been speaking of religious devotion, but there are numerous figureheads and organizations which serve exactly the same function. Political parties or political beliefs are vociferously defended by devotees as being the repository of ultimate truth. Diet fanatics will attribute healing properties to certain dietary truths, paying homage at the feet of whole-wheat bread or organic vegetables. They serve a purpose, to allay the fear of accepting that there is no higher authority than ourselves.

The people who believe in higher authorities are those who as children have been told, usually indirectly and therefore more powerfully, that the world is unsafe. They are never encouraged to believe that they are powerful enough to care for themselves, and never have the reins of self-responsibility handed to them in a safe and caring way, as they become capable of taking them. They are encouraged to remain under the influence of others, sometimes parents, sometimes the church, or are left to find their own godhead. If they are angry with parents, they'll pick a belief as visibly removed from that of their parents as possible, for example, if the parents are Christian, they may be fervent Hare Krishnas. In reality they have adopted the parental belief system, that is, it's necessary to believe in something more strongly than you believe in yourself. This recreates their experience of childhood, when they were unable to look after themselves. To maintain it forever is to always deny our own power over fate, which is the traditional illness position. Lived like this, life is at least homogeneous. There's no need to change just because we're now adults. It's consistent and, above all, it's safe. It clearly suits many people.

The alternative is to regard life as consisting of two general phases. The first phase is childhood, a period of diminished responsibility. The second is adulthood, the period of full responsibility. In the first phase our parents are the ultimate authority we know. As grown-ups we are the ultimate authority, although the law may frustrate us. We are faced, in this model, with two changes, just as there are two phases. The first change we make is to adapt to our parents' wishes. We become either what they want us to be or its opposite. Either way we have still modified our behavior in response to our parents' demands. That's the first change we make. The second change is the change back. Having modified our thoughts, feelings and behaviors out of necessity in childhood, we now change back to thinking, feeling and behaving as we, our new parent figures, want. To do this we need to drop those parts of our childhood conditioning that we adopted for safety, but which we no longer require. We no longer need a figurehead to keep us safe or alive. We are free. That's the second change, the change back. Perhaps that's what Jesus Christ meant when he said, "Else ye turn and become as little children, ye shall not enter the kingdom of heaven."

There's a transition period between the first and second phases that occurs usually between adolescence and young adulthood. When parents are aware of handing responsibility to their children, or do so intuitively, then the transition phase will be successfully accomplished with a minimum of trauma. There will be plenty of adjustments for the new adult to make, but he'll have the confidence and skills to handle them with ease. He will believe in his ability to take whatever steps will benefit him most. He'll have little need for illness to help him through this phase.

For those of us who didn't get what we wanted in childhood and who were forced to adapt more of our own wants to meet parent's needs, there are other methods available to us to make the change back. It may be frightening, because the level of adaptation may have been so great that we don't know what it's like to be just what we want, to be ourselves, to be free. We can't remember or conceive of such a state. We may not be motivated to try for it unless the pain of our present circumstances becomes too great. Illness may be one of those motivating factors. It may feel much safer to accept a level of discomfort and try to ignore it, using work, family, politics or religion. We may not want to address ourselves to the possibility of dropping our defenses and risking the unknown. We may have carved out a niche of caring that, despite needing the occasional sinus attack to keep it operational, serves us well. We settle for it. For those intrepid souls who reach for the sky, psychotherapy, meditation, religion, fanaticism of any kind, a guru or a friend may serve to keep us safe through the transition period between dependence on parents and dependence on self. We are like a caterpillar entering the cocoon from which, if it is to achieve its life destiny, it must emerge. To emerge from this phase is to drop the transitional belief system and to create one of our own. The psychotherapy is no longer relevant, the guru's trip becomes his own. We reject him with love. We are free.

IV

THE PREVENTION OF ILLNESS AND THE CREATION OF WELLNESS

19

Levels of Prevention

Prevention has several components. An illness that has taken hold may be prevented from becoming worse. An illness that has been removed completely may be prevented from recurring. An adult may prevent illnesses from which other members of her family have suffered by taking preventive measures. She may elect to do this at any time in her life. Lastly, and I think the aspect of prevention that has been virtually ignored, is the prevention of illness in children and adults by preventive or healthy parenting. This involves relating to our children in such a way as to encourage wellness and to discourage the need for illness. To do this would significantly alter medical practice. Meanwhile, let us look at those measures, which we adults, who perhaps were not taught how to avoid illness, can take for ourselves now.

In previous chapters I have described how we give ourselves illnesses, which confirm early childhood decisions about ourselves, our parents and the world. Rather than face the fear of doing things differently,

we choose to continue with the old beliefs and behaviors, even though they're damaging to our psyche
and our bodies. In this way illness takes care of our
greatest fears and may be regarded as an ego defense
mechanism. If we are prepared to risk being scared,
we can investigate the origins of our disease and learn
what we can do to remove it. This may vary from
changing jobs to admitting and expressing (indirectly)
the anger towards our father for deserting us. Having
learned the cause of the illness, that is, why we have
decided at that time to become sick, we then choose
whether to remove it or not. Both choices, taken with
awareness and responsibility, are equally valid. For
example, we may choose to understand why we've
made ourselves ill, choose not to proceed with those
behaviors that would make the condition worse and
choose to retain the conditioning that maintains the
disease. There are many good reasons for adopting this
attitude, and in practice many people choose this level
of prevention. Some of these reasons include financial
commitments, family responsibilites or, most often,
the fear of loss of love. An example follows.

A thirty-year-old woman supporting her three children consulted me complaining of pelvic inflammatory
disease, a long-term problem she had suffered since
the break-up of her marriage three years ago. She'd
been given eight courses of various antibiotics in that
time, all administered by a gynecologist in the hope of
settling the inflammation. The pain lessened for a
while, then recurred. Hormones, in the form of various
brands of the contraceptive pill, were also tried.
    We established that she felt guilty about depriving
her children of their father. She'd had a brief affair
and took responsibility for the ensuing break-up of her

marriage. When I suggested to her that her pelvic inflammatory disease would improve if she slowed down at work, she began to cry and said that since it was her fault that the children were without a father, the least she could do was to insure they didn't want for anything material. She was not prepared to reduce her working hours. She was prepared, however, to stop feeling guilty at having an affair, realizing that it was a symptom of the marriage, rather than the cause of the divorce, and to stop taking responsibility for the action of her previous husband. In particular she stopped regarding her sexual infidelity as the reason for all her problems. The disease settled and, since she didn't take a rest, continued in a mild form for the next year. In this case the woman arrested her disease and prevented it from worsening.

This example can be extended to cover the second type of prevention, preventing the recurrence of a disease that the client had removed completely. If the woman with the pelvic inflammatory disease had taken a vacation or rested more often, as well as stopping feeling guilty, she would have stopped inflaming her own sexual organs and her condition would have resolved. If she was prepared to become aware of those times in childhood when she decided, in response to her father, that she was responsible for men leaving her and that it was because of her sexuality, she might cure her disease forever. This would involve disowning the responsibility she took for her mother's jealousy of the way in which her father cared for her. She was not to blame for her father leaving home, despite her mother's insinuations, and to be loved she need no longer feel guilty as she decided to then. She had, of course, repeated these exact conditions in her own life, which demonstrates the power of scripting, or the fear of loss of parental love. If she marries a man who will not leave her, will not hold her responsible for his own feelings, and who's happy to tell her how wonderfully sexy she is, she'll have resolved the matter. She may, of course, resolve it in other ways.

As adults, we can improve the general quality of our health in non-specific ways. We can practice general prevention, and by so doing avoid degenerative diseases, or perhaps prevent those diseases that our family histories almost guaranteed we would contract. Every member of a family over fifty may have suffered from arthritis, for example. In practicing this sort of prevention, we take note of such factors as diet, lifestyle, recreation, exercise, spirituality, sleep patterns, rest, interests, retirement planning, meditative practices, and interpersonal and family relationships. These are the general considerations.

I have dealt with the topic of preventive diet before. The "diet of best chance," "prudent diet," "Long-term general diet" and "preventive diet" are all the same thing. This, I took pains to point out, was completely different from "remedial diet," which is the acute treatment of specific disease in specific individuals by altering their physiology and psychology using constantly changing diets. I will briefly discuss the other factors in general prevention before examining the area of disease avoidance I consider most important—preventive or healthy parenting.

The general consensus appears to be that one who eats a prudent diet, sleeps between six and ten hours a night so as to awake refreshed, and takes an amount of exercise that will keep the heart and lungs active, is the happiest and healthiest. Such a person will have a loving spouse, between two and three well-adjusted, loving children, have interests outside the home, be intellectually stimulated and stimulating, have great sex at least three times a week and will be unafraid to masturbate or be known to masturbate. In her life there will be a fine balance of commitment, rest and recreation. Spiritually she will be both surrendered and flexible, perhaps a member of the Christian church or interested in Buddhism or meditation. Others will notice her inner peace. She will be receptive to the political and social troubles of our times, have the strength to change those things she can, and the wisdom to accept those she can't. She'll be both existentially content and continually evolving as a personality. Above all she will accept her own power to do as she wishes, while both considering others and not accepting their burdens as her own. Among her friends will be soul mates, perhaps one or two, up to four close friends and a number of acquaintances with whom she spends a little time. She has learned to live with paradox.

What was your reaction to the above cameo? Were you wishing you were there, not believing some or much of it to be possible, angry at not being like this woman, positively nauseated by the thought of it, thinking it was a hoax, wanting some of it for you but rejecting other aspects of it, not wanting any of it, confused about what you do want, seeing it as idyllic, scared that you may never make it, dismissing it as a hippie plot to return to peace, love and sisterhood, sad that you have a long way to go, resigned to mediocrity, wanting to forget the whole thing, angry that Buddha and Jesus Christ were mentioned as equals, wondering if it's the same for a man, or wanting to adopt it as a good way to be?

Is your response some of the above, all of the above, or none of the above?

The likelihood is that you already have some of

those things, are in the process of acquiring others and are disinterested in the remainder. By such an exercise it's possible to see that a general description of health and happiness in one fictitious person actually describes no one. This doesn't mean that no one has achieved that degree of fulfillment, but that fulfillment, health and happiness are different things to different people. That's hardly a shattering statement. We're all aware that we have quite different tastes, dislikes and aspirations from those of our neighbors, even our spouses, and that it causes us no problem. Few of us would welcome changing so that we all became the same. If we apply this same reasoning to health, it becomes clear that some aspects of my body and mind function, which I regard as a disease (am uneasy about) will be regarded by some readers as a minor inconvenience or of no significance. Certainly they wouldn't bother to do anything about it, whereas I'm searching for the way and the will to change it. Similarly, conditions from which you and I both suffer and which are of great concern to you may be of no importance to me. In addition, we all forgo a degree of health in order to achieve other things. A woman supporting her children may have dermatitis of the hands from the need to do extra cleaning, and accept that. To another woman that would be intolerable. I've spent most of the past thirty summers on the beach surfing. To experience the exhilaration, the fear and the triumph of riding waves is important to me, and I'm prepared to accept the premature aging and drying of my skin, which is an inevitable consequence of such an activity. I take the precautions I can, but I am not prepared to stay indoors just because my blond complexion evolved in milder, less sunny climates than Australia, where I was born and have lived all my life.

I take full responsibility for that decision, knowing that I have no intention of suffering from it.

It's because we all differ so much that general recommendations are, at best, of little use. This makes real nonsense of the fanatics reported in newspapers who have decided that we would all eat fish and no red meat, or we should all play squash or handball, or that we should all sleep from 10:00 p.m. until 6:00 a.m. They've also decided for us that we shouldn't smoke, that we need a blood test for cancer every year and that organic vegetables are the only way of keeping our bodies free of pollutants. What they really mean is that they need to eat organic vegetables and to not smoke, because if they didn't, then they would be imbalanced. It has, of course, nothing to do with us. Their effort to convert others to their way of thinking is for their own benefit. Often they are seeking approval for their discovery and that's not dishonorable. People get acknowledged the best way they can. What it means for us, the readers, is that we accept only those theories and practices that agree with our own assessment. From time to time, in order to advance, we may need to risk those old assessments but we needn't take anyone else's word for it. We can listen. We can decide.

20

Healthy Parenting

I believe that the most important aspect of preventive medicine, or health promotion, is preventive parenting. This refers to the messages parents give their children in the early years (the first six are the most important) that shape the child's personality. These years are most important because young children are the most vulnerable and the most impressionable. If children are raised to be autonomous, they won't need major illness. What does being autonomous involve?

Autonomy, according to Berne in *Games People Play*, has three components: awareness, spontaneity and intimacy. Awareness has two components: sensory awareness, which means intact taste, touch, sight, smell and hearing; and psychological clarity. Spontaneity refers to the willingness to feel joy, anger, sadness and fear, and to express them. Intimacy refers to loving and being loved in warm, caring and satisfying transactions. These three characteristics are considerations of both parenting and therapy.

In Chapter 2—The Childhood Basis of Disease, I discussed the ways in which the injunctions and the drivers were acted upon by children, with the subsequent development of disease, while the permissions and the allowers promoted autonomy and health.

The most important of the permissions is "exist." A child who's uncertain whether her parents wanted her will substantially modify her behavior in order to be allowed (as she sees it) to remain alive. These modifications cause disease in the short and long terms via mechanisms that have been elaborated elsewhere. The injunctions and the drivers are modifications of the right to exist; for example, in the case of the injunction "don't be a girl," it's OK for you to exist providing you aren't a girl. Or in the case of the driver "be strong," it's OK for you to exist only as long as you're strong. A child who believes that one or both parents are not totally happy with her being alive will begin life on a shaky foundation. Someone who never really believes that she has an unqualified right to exist will not continually influence her own body positively, and her physique will end up an accurate reflection of her fears and insecurities. Illness is guaranteed.

The first step in preventive parenting, or more accurately healthy parenting, is to affirm and reaffirm the right of children to be alive. Parents will feel comfortable in doing this in their own ways. The overall message will be the equivalent of "Sweetheart, I love you, and I love having you around." If this is repeated frequently in the early years, and said at impromptu times when the child has done absolutely nothing to "deserve" it (that is, it was totally unsolicited) then the child will believe that truly she's a joy to her parents and that they want her. Needless to say, the child will detect any falseness in this and other messages she receives, so there's no point in lying to her. Better to say nothing, or tell the truth if you're feeling like stroking her. Body language, voice intonation, and of course facial expression will tell the child, well before she has acquired language, what is meant. If the words are different from the way they are expressed, children will believe their own interpretation. A child whose parents have told her they love her, but did things that would suggest otherwise, will not be convinced by the words. She'll end up not trusting anything she's told and be very confused indeed. If the parents don't want the child and regret her existence, then it is better to adopt her out to someone who will love and cherish her. If that opportunity has passed, then I believe the child will be better off if she's not lied to. There's no point in telling her that she's not wanted, she'll pick that up anyway, but it will be less damaging in the long run to be a real parent, however unloving, than a false parent. It will be painful, but she can work through it later.

More common than parents who don't want their children are parents who love their children but don't tell them. For example, many men believe that to tell children they are loved is to be an unmanly father and that if the child is a boy, such a statement is unbecoming. They may be afraid of telling their daughters, perhaps equating love with sexual intimacy. They believe that children can be spoiled by love, or demonstrated love. I don't agree with them but I respect their own personal need to withhold the verbal affirmation of their love. They do this because of their own fears and not for the reason they usually give, which is that it's good for the children. I encourage them to resolve their fear and to start stroking their children, both verbally and physically, for I know from experience that their children will be much healthier, knowing and hearing they are loved.

Feeling loved is not the same as being inconsiderate of others, or believing that you can always have your own way. Many parents believe that to continually reaffirm their love for their kids by telling them so and hugging them will mean the kids grow up to be demanding monsters. On the contrary, it's much easier and more effective to say, "You can't have that because we don't have the money," in a loving way (that is "It's OK to ask; you can't have it, and I love you") than to be refusing children who ask for things out of the frustration of not knowing whether they're loved or not. They ask in anger. The anger is not at being refused what they want but at not feeling loved. The former is a short-lived disappointment, the latter an ever-increasing antagonism that only love can cure. Those children who appear obnoxious, arrogant or spoiled are protesting at the way in which they have been bought off by parents willing to indulge their every whim, rather than love them for what they are. They are responding to a need in the parent, a need that the children are in no way capable of satisfying. They struggle to do it, however, in their quest for survival. A spoiled child may be the result of parents so in need themselves that they desperately long for their child to love them and try to buy that love. The child responds with anger at this blackmail, as she loves her parents anyway, and recognizes the ulterior message to her, which is that her love is not good enough to satisfy her parents. This contrasts with the child who is convinced of her parents' love, and is under no obligation to love them back in a particular way. Children will love parents without having to be coaxed into it. Love doesn't cause spoiled children, it cures them.

The other permissions and allowers naturally follow the unqualified right to exist. In fact they are the unqualified right to exist. Look at these a moment (go back to page 32), and ask yourself about you and your children; do you encourage them to feel their emotions, cry when they're sad, get angry at you when you do something they don't like, or do you use your physical power and greater intellect to keep them subservient? When you've asked yourself that question, you might ask whether the pattern of your own childhood is not repeating itself, and remind yourself how you felt about it at the time. If you are like the rest of us, the likelihood is that you'll have repeated some of your own childhood messages to your own children, even though some of them were distressing to you at the time. Or you may have decided in childhood that when you had kids, you were sure you weren't going to make your kids go through what you went through. You might be telling your kids that you love them, just as you wished your parents had told you, allowing your daughter to become womanly and sexy, just as you wished you'd been allowed to, letting your boy cry as you were encouraged not to. Will you consider giving yourself the same caring permissions you're giving your kids? After all, you're now your own parent, as well as theirs.

If children are given the sorts of affirmations I've been speaking of, their need for illness will be reduced. If illness is regarded as a defense mechanism, and the individual has little need to be defended, then she'll have little need for illness. Because we are all defended to some degree, and because we are living in an hostile environment, we all suffer intermittently.

Pollutants in the form of colorings, flavorings, preservatives, car fumes, industrial fallout, microwaves, genetics, noise, tension in children and their parents, chlorinated water, excessive dairy products, poor bowel function and a lack of fresh green vegetables all play a part in the development of upper respiratory tract infections in children. They are almost inevitable, even in children who are loved. When the first stage of prevention, health-promoting parenting, fails to prevent the development of disease, we need to isolate those factors that are maintaining it or making it worse. This prevents future, more severe attacks from occurring by minimizing the influence of those factors beyond our control, and eliminating those under our control. We can minimize the effect of those factors out of our control by not adding to them.

When a child develops an infection, or more often an inflammation, her immediate needs must be attended to by her parents. She is rested, fed a remedial diet, counseled about problems and about future lifestyle, and given the same amount of caring as if she were well. The illness does not attract increased parental energy and support. To do that simply guarantess its repetition. Particularly if brothers and sisters demand equal attention from the parents, children will be very quick to seize upon any activity, which increases their share of the parental caring. Illness is a favorite. Initially it may be necessary to give the child less caring than if she were well in order to encourage her to change her illness pattern, although this may result in attention-seeking behavior equally as undesirable as the disease. Future attacks may jeopardize the long-term health of the child and strong immediate measures may be required. At the same time as the patient is offered minimal caring, other children in the family may be stroked and congratulated on keeping themselves well. Wellness is therefore rewarded, illness is not. Children respond very quickly to a change in the reward system and are very aware of its ramifications, as demonstrated by the five-year-old client of mine overheard by his parents as he pointed out to his three-year-old sister: "If you want Mommy to look after you, just get sick, that's what I do." When children come into my office and one member of the family is ill, I am careful to pay equal attention to the healthy. Since some of them like coming to see me, I arrange times for them to visit when they are well. They begin replacing illness with wellness.

It will often be necessary for parents to examine and change their own patterns of illness if they want their children to become well. There's little point in parents complaining about seven-year-old Mary always having stomach cramps and staying away from school before an exam when the mother takes to bed with an aspirin or two when she's feeling tense. Similarly, little Freddie's foot is unlikely to improve enough to allow him to take part in sports lessons while his father is still at home with a "bad back." We are creating the illness patterns of our children every time we suffer from an illness ourselves. We can minimize the effects of this modeling by being truthful about what's happening to us—"Son, when I was your age I lost my father in a car accident. Since then I get asthma when I'm scared about something and, as you know, right now I'm in line for this promotion and it's scaring me a little. I'm not sure why I hang onto the asthma, but I do know only I can remove it. As for you, well, you can decide to be well." By owning our power to be well or ill, we model that for our offspring.

Paradoxically, permitting illness is a necessary part of promoting wellness. If we're overzealous about discouraging illness in children we may be inadvertently telling them to not look after themselves. Illness is a legitimate way of meeting needs, and when we attempt to discourage it on the grounds that it causes long-term harm to our bodies, we need to be very sure that we are not telling children that they're not OK because they've chosen illness to meet their needs. Rather we can isolate the need, attend to that part of it which is our responsibility as a parent, and teach our children to take care of themselves by asking for what they want if they are unable to provide it themselves. As support for this, we need, of course, to be willing to provide the caring in other ways. We support them for doing something to improve their lives, while recommending a less damaging way of going about it. Consider the following:

"Why aren't you at school today, David?"

"I hurt my knee."

"How did you do that?"

"Playing football."

"What's on at school today, anything special?"

"Just another football match, that's all."

"Don't you want to play?"

"No. It's too rough. Peter Smith is a big bully, and Tom's always after me, he's about twice as big as me."

"Don't play if you don't want to."

"Then Tom's father'll call me a sissy. He reckons only girls don't play football."

"Are there others who don't play?"

"Sure, lots of 'em."

"Are they sissies?"

"No."

"It's OK by me if you don't play football. I used to love playing tennis."

Taking care of children's needs and then handing responsibility to them when they're capable of taking

it is an art. It's also one of the main factors in the creation of wellness, or the prevention of illness. How
might we go about this?

Children begin acquiring skills at a very early age.
By the age of six months they're able to hold objects
in their hands and pick up those things they've
dropped, provided they can reach them. They may not
be able to crawl or sit properly at this stage. The art
of letting them do things of which they're capable or
that they want to practice begins in infancy. When the
child drops an object that is of interest to her and her
hand control is sufficiently developed to enable her to
pick it up, let her. By so doing the child develops the
skill, becomes surer that she can get the things she
wants, confirms her belief that her parents are interested in her developing skills, believes that it's OK
to do things for herself, and continues to mature. At
six months she'll need help to be placed where she can
retrieve the object, and by a parent putting her there
and letting her pick it up, she learns about asking for
help and receiving it. She grows safe in the belief that
she will be permitted to benefit herself when she's
able and receive help when she needs it. She reckons
the world to be a safe, caring place.

A child who lets her mother or father know that
she's interested in an object by reaching for it or by
making a noise, and receives no help in getting it, will
start believing that she has little power over her life;
she hasn't the skills to do it herself and nobody seems
interested in helping her. If this happens often
enough, she resigns herself to powerlessness. She may
also make the decision that she's helpless and loveless.
I have outlined previously how these feelings soon express themselves in physical disease.

Alternatively, a child who has her needs attended
to but is not allowed to help herself, that is, she wants

the object, and although capable of picking it up, has it repeatedly picked up for her, understands that her needs will be met, but probably decides there's something scary about meeting them herself. Such a child grows up feeling loved but incapable. The world is safe only as long as someone else is about to take care of things. She accepts her parents' fears about life being dangerous. As an adult she will be tempted to become ill to be cared for, as this option is condoned by society.

I have described a six-month-old infant, but the process of striking a balance between caring for children and letting them care for themselves occurs between birth and when the offspring leave home, and even after that. As a child becomes older, another hazard arises: encouraging or even forcing children to take care of themselves and others (usually parents) before they're able. This creates enormous anxiety in the child, and usually means she suppresses her own needs and feelings in favor of those expected of her. Eventually, the little kid inside her becomes exhausted from the burden and collapses, physically and mentally. This may happen at any age, and until it does, these people are often bastions of self-responsibility and caring for others. I have even known physicians of community standing who were heroin addicts. Therapy involves the client's own grown-up taking care of her own little kid. Prevention involves having expectations of our children that they are old enough to handle.

As children become teenagers, the task of steering a middle course becomes seemingly impossible, at times, with the need of the teenager to rebel and the influence of peer groups and societal messages in conflict with those of the parents. It has little to do with prevention of illness, as the crucial period for estab-

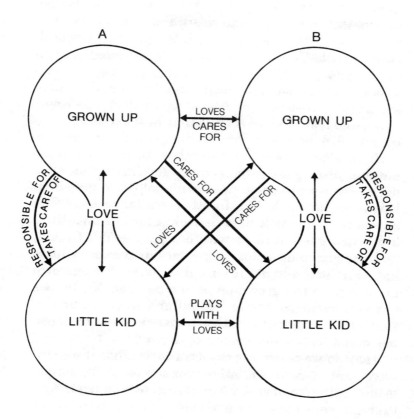

lishing a pattern of caring and safety and encouraging self-responsibility is accomplished before the age of ten. In later years it is refined.

Another component of healthy parenting is teaching children to pick someone with whom they'll be happy to spend their lives. Indirectly this will prohibit illness by meeting needs before the need for illness becomes necessary. I have the following concept of marriage. I refer here to a partnership between two people in love who are of opposite sexes, the same sex, bound by law or by private contract, intending to have children or not. The partners may be regarded as two adults with two children in their charge. The two little kids are, of course, their own internal kids. The little kid in us represents our needs, wants, loves, feelings, hopes and fears; the part of us that needs protection to be provided by the grown-up part. In a partnership, each grown-up takes responsibility for her own little kid and also takes responsibility for finding another person who's grown-up who will help her grown-up look after her little kid. In other words, we each find a grown-up who will help us look after our own little kid. Our little kid plays with our partner's little kid, and our grown-up helps look after our partner's little kid. Our little kid doesn't need to look after our own grown-up, or the grown-up of our partner. Nor do we ask our partner's kid to look after our grown-up. By such an arrangement, each partner remains responsible, cared for, caring, loving and loved.

How do we teach our children to do this? If we ourselves are in such a relationship, it's easy. We simply model being in love by simultaneously having fun, taking care of ourselves and caring for our partner. At the same time we adopt the attitude to our children's needs as described previously. If we aren't in such a relationship, it's more difficult. We may use metaphor or storytelling and, as the child becomes more able to understand, explain our position directly. We can place our children in the company of adults who enjoy a partnership that does model the behavior, and we can comment favorably upon the behavior of others to whom the child has access. We can allow the child to choose differently from ourselves by recalling the allowers and permissions mentioned previously. Above all, as they leave childhood we can confirm the love we had, and have, for them.

Lastly, in healthy parenting we can instruct our children in those lifestyles, eating habits, etcetera, which we have found to be helpful for us, and make available information, which we haven't tried or used ourselves, but which we feel may be of value. We can encourage an attitude within the child of respect for her own individuality and the idea that decisions about herself will ultimately need to be her own. As she is different from every other person on the planet, those decisions will be necessarily unique and untried. She will be prepared for the risk.

21

At Your Invitation Only

Whenever I read a psychotherapy book, or attend a lecture by a fellow therapist, I constantly modify what's being said with my perception of who's saying it. My assessment will be based on my observation of his body language, his general state of anxiety, the way he relates to his spouse, his use of language, his major representational system, and so on. I have previously discussed in great detail diagnosis by observation. As the personality of the therapist emerges, what he's really saying becomes clearer, and I'm able to assess its relevance for me. I use my skills of observation to sift rapidly through an otherwise formidable amount of theory about health and healing. All theory arises within the theorist's own experience. That may sound obvious, but if we use that maxim, some well-accepted theories and practices become recognizable for what they really are—an individual writing not of some universal truth, but of himself. Medicine abounds with "scientific" hypotheses, which are statistically valid one year and "disproven" the next.

For the brief period of their acceptance by the "scientific" fraternity, they are the only truth, maintained if need be by the scurrilous deposition of alternative views. Then someone, working from his own internal needs as did his predecessor, discovers something that is "truer," that is, more fulfilling of both his own needs and the needs of those responsible for accrediting new theories and practices.

Man interprets what he sees, rather than describes it. Red to me is a collection of colors that I have seen over the years, which were called red by my parents and others. To you, red will be almost the same, but not quite, since your experience will have been different. If we both saw a color that was borderline red, then it's likely we would differ as to what we called it—I would say "sort of red" and you "sort of yellow." Similarly, an individual living in Ireland all his life has a quite different notion of what constitutes "green" flora than does someone living in Australia. A tree described as "green" by the Australian would be considered "gray" by the Irishman. Hardly scientific. In a similar manner, patients are diagnosed and treated differently by different practitioners. For example, I believe that if an individual is not having sex (either intercourse or masturbation), that's imbalance. My treatment of that person will take that into account. Another practitioner may view that as contentment, and call it balance. The client concerned will be attracted to me because of my views, or will reject my approach and go elsewhere. No practitioner has a mortgage on the truth. There is no truth, simply a subjective, biased interpretation of unverifiable, fluctuating data. The interpretation the client accepts will be the interpretation that suits him at that time. It will be the one with which he is most comfortable (or least afraid). Later he may be prepared to risk more, and increase his level of discomfort in order to achieve something he considers important. Then he may need to change practitioners. Any investment I have in him accepting my ideas about his condition will ultimately stand in the way of his resolving his problem, and he must realize that. If he doesn't want to take responsibility for himself, he'll invite my interpretation and take it as gospel, rather than use it to clarify his own beliefs. By so doing he hopes I'll relieve him of the burden of looking after himself. The value to me in being regarded as fallible by the client is that I don't have to pretend to look after him.

I believe that the energy for a hypothesis comes partly from a denial of its opposite. If I'm afraid to express my emotions, then I'm likely to develop a treatment modality that is intellectually orientated and be able to "prove" that expressing emotions is of little value in psychotherapy. The more strident I am about my beliefs the more likely I am to be afraid of their opposites. When I campaign long and hard for the death penalty for murder, I am denying the part of me that would murder. Much bigotry has its roots in the fact that the proponent of a viewpoint fears he is the very thing he finds so abhorrent. None of this would matter so much if it weren't essential, in order to deny the fear, that some people attempt to inflict their attitudes on others. In such a way I'm denied seeing and hearing what I deem to be healthy for me because a censor, afraid of his own lasciviousness needs to believe he knows what's best for me. He imagines my impurity as a way of denying his own. My way of life is affected by others needing to justify their own actions taken as they are, not in the light of knowledge and objectivity, but in the service of their fears. Pity those who trap themselves in the medical system, are scared to abscond, and who wake up without their gallbladders. They will get little comfort from the knowledge that they have helped a surgeon stave off his fear that there was a less traumatic way to cure the patient.

Current medical practice may be regarded as the result of the medical profession and the public combining to defend themselves against the fear of self-exposure and alternative views. It has little concern for those theories and practices that could keep most people free of physical and mental disease. The more mechanistic and strident the conservative element in the medical profession becomes, the more afraid they are. Change, flexibility and human concerns become increasingly dismissed in favor of spending large amounts of money to shore up a system that was never effective in curing people. It does, however, temporarily allay the feelings of impotence of those claiming responsibility for the health of others. The alternative is self-responsibility. Some doctors and members of the public may not like it, for it means stopping telling people what they should do, and letting them do what is right for them. Bureaucracies, like medical hierarchies, fail to survive when they are no longer funded by fear.

So too is this book a reflection of both my aspirations and my fears. That I should propose self-responsiblity for you all comes from my reluctance to accept my own, or my unwillingness to trust others. Am I not, by writing this book, seeking your tacit approval for my ideas and indirectly your admiration for me? Do I only feel safe if I know that you, my public, loves me? I am both yearning for you to need my advice and caring, and angry that I put myself in a position of taking care of your needs. Like most doctors, I have been raised to care for others, and I do it very well. From the paradox of my feelings, and the honing of my perceptions and interpretations in childhood, comes my therapy. I cannot tell you what to do, because I do not know. What I can tell you is what I have found in living my life up to this point in time. I am subjective and my conclusions constantly change. Therein lies their value. You can read them, allow them to affect you, dream about them and ultimately discard them in favor of your own immediate truth.

That people who intend becoming well must decide for themselves is for many a bitter pill to swallow. We all twist and turn in order to avoid that realization, searching often all our lives to find someone or something to take care of us. And yet there's a part of us that is continually rejecting advice from authorities, even after we have expended much effort in obtaining it. Clients almost seduce doctors into advising them, promising to be good, reliable patients, "I'll do anything to get rid of it, Doctor," only to dismiss the recommendations. I have argued before that this well-recognized phenomenon is often in the service of continuing the illness, a part of the contract between the patient and his practitioner. But there's another component to it as well. We encourage a prophet to promote his views, give him credence, patronize his practice, spread the word of his wonderful cures and lure him into believing he's infallible. We promote him to a position of power, often forgiving minor transgressions of his stated aims along the way. He becomes a figurehead, and people look to him for guidance. He cannot assume power over people, or over their views—they must give it to him. Secretly people regard him as a fool, though they take care until the time is right to not publicize their view. And then he stumbles, often with the help of someone apparently sympathetic but secretly aspiring to his position, but mostly because he can no longer stand the solitude and fear of being top dog. His fall from power is often dramatic, aided by scandal of some sort. We strip him of his power exactly as we gave it to him, musing in his passing at what possessed him to make the oldest mistake on earth. We have made him a fool. The sorrow of the occasion is tempered by memories of the early dream, when we hope he would save us. Soon both sorrow and memories are lost beneath the crushing inevitability of his demise. We settle back to defending ourselves against the realization of our own aloneness, quietly plotting to whom we'll next give the mantle of hero. Before long he appears.

We do this in the hope of avoiding responsibility. Our fear is that we're not good enough, since we didn't attract the perfect love and caring we hoped for as children. We are terrified that even if we risk changing that won't be good enough to please the new parents, just as we weren't good enough to please the original ones. Better to stay helpless, loveless, hopeless and ill; then we may at least attract caring.

CONCEPTS OF HEALING

Many people have concerned themselves with the nature of the healing force. It's the same as the illness force, coming from within the client. That part of the client, which is prepared to accept responsiblity for having caused the illness can now take responsibility for curing it. If 85 percent of illness is acknowledged as self-caused, the same 85 percent becomes available for self-cure. Wow, I can cure 85 percent of my illness myself! If factors beyond the individual's control are deemed to have caused 85 percent of the illness, only 15 percent becomes available for self-cure. We then put ourselves in the hands of an expert, relying upon him to cure the remaining 85 percent of our illness. This is a sobering thought in view of the fact that he'll be looking after his interests first and ours, if we're lucky, second. By being willing to accept a large portion of our disease as of our making, created in order to take care of ourselves best, we make available an equally large portion about which we can choose to do something. This makes us responsible and in control of our own healing process. It doesn't matter what other people, experts or friends, regard as a reasonable percentage of the disease to acknowledge as our own. We can vary the percentage according to how much we want to take responsibility for ourselves at any time. Understanding that we have made ourselves ill in order to care for ourselves, and to congratulate ourselves on so doing, is an early step to feeling good about saying, "Yes, I made myself ill, and now I choose to make myself well."

Taking responsiblity for the future requires that we take responsiblity for the past. That means accepting that even though we were in a position where we had few options, our reactions were our own. When we can accept the old hurts, we can drop them and our old anger. We changed the way we were in order to survive. Now we must change back in order to survive. These are the two changes of life. The first was made under duress and with few or no options. The second change, the change back, is entirely up to us. We need not undergo the laborious process of altering every decision we've taken. Why should we? We're happy enough with the very large part of us. There may be a few of our personal idiosyncracies that result in us

not getting what we want. Some of these will be causing illness. The change back to the way we were need
not be an agonizing process.

Watch a weight-lifter. Watch his face as he contem-
plates the lift, wondering if he'll make it. Watch his
struggle and the stress on his frame as he uses every
fiber of his body to effect the lift, drawing on his hours
of physical and mental training. Notice the hope and
the fear as he reaches upwards in the last final thrust.
See the exhilaration on his face as he feels the
straightening of his arms as he achieves his goal. See
his moment of peace and fulfillment as he walks from
beneath his weight and sees it crash effortlessly into
the mat.

We have struggled to lift a large and cumbersome
burden onto our shoulders because we were told to. It
took us about six years of hard labor, lifting it bit by
bit. We have struggled to live while carrying it
around. Our back hurts and our head aches. We
daren't lean forward and we daren't lean back. We
needn't lower it inch by inch as we raised it. We
needn't consider each painful decision we took all
those years ago as we were raising it. We needn't
break our backs lowering it as we lifted it. We can
walk from under it. It will fall to the ground with no
effort and with no pain. We can drop it.

As a therapist, I cast myself in the role of, and am
cast in the role of, a surrogate parent. We all use surrogate parents until we no longer need them. Whenever clients consult therapists, transference occurs.
When the client no longer needs a surrogate parent in
order to feel safe, he will no longer need to attend the
therapist. That's cure. This may be a problem for a
therapist who only feels safe when he's looking after
people. He may not regard the client curing himself

and leaving therapy to be in his (the therapist's) interests. He may be tempted to maintain the transference and counter-transference, and keep the client in therapy. This happens in psychotherapy more often than therapists care to admit. Therapists are cast by clients into roles purely for the benefit of the client's needs ("You're wonderful, Doctor") and they in turn are cast as clients ("I can fix you") for the benefit of therapists. This can be a pitfall of therapy, as neither the client nor the doctor ever leaves it.

THE ILLNESS CYCLE

If childhood didn't provide an environment in which to learn that we were loved, and didn't equip us for adulthood by a gradual and safe handing over of the responsibility of looking after ourselves, we tend to look for surrogate parents to cover the transition period between leaving home and being self-responsible. In this period people seek therapy, among other things. I'm of the belief that this is a period of transition, which for the future peace of mind of all of us who needed therapy, we must pass through.

There's an added bonus to walking away from this transition period and dropping therapy. It comes in the form of effective partner selection. If we select a partner while we are in the transition period of diminished personal responsibility, our partner will be chosen as a surrogate parent. He will only be available if he's in the same stage, that is, of denying that people are responsible for themselves. He expresses this belief by taking care of his partner. Although partners respond differently, one taking care of, the other being cared for, they have the same belief system. These partnerships last only as long as both partners remain in the transition phase. When one moves on, the other will feel unsafe. They'll often move along together, in which case they report a growing and maturing of their relationship. If one partner refuses, through fear, to take responsiblity for himself, and the other moves through the transition phase, the relationship collapses. Alternatively, two people who form a partnership, both from a position of self-responsiblity, will be able to choose their partners unshackled by the above complications. They are likely to make wiser choices.

One of the major reasons a client attends a practitioner is to have his needs recognized. If a busy doctor spends five or ten minutes with the patient, half of this time with his head buried in the drug compendium searching for the latest remedy, the patient is very likely to go away feeling that he's been dealt with perfunctorily. The treatment prescribed may be enough to relieve his symptoms, but the underlying psychological states have not been dealt with and, since they are a major component of any illness, the condition is unlikely to resolve. The client often becomes angry at such a dismissal of his real needs and, as many a doctor finds out, makes himself worse and then threatens to sue for negligence. Those practitioners who spend more time with clients tend to be sued less. Sometimes the client only needs to be seen for a short time, but these are rare. Repeat of a drug prescription is an example. However, if he's wanting a repeat prescription, it would appear that both parties have settled for palliative (non-curative) treatment, and a review is perhaps warranted. If the client has a new complaint, one hour is the minimum time necessary to establish the client's needs, how the complaint is meeting those needs and what alternative options are available. The five-minute consultation, followed by the routine prescription of a drug, is virtually the only medicine practiced by the vast majority of doctors. This reflects, of course, the vast majority of people's wishes.

Unless a consultation occupies a substantial amount of time, the doctor and the client never enter the trance state necessary for comprehension and cure of the problem. When I'm in the middle of an interview with a client and the telephone rings, I become aware of just how deeply in trance I am. I've been occupied totally by what he's saying and my observation of how he's saying it. I'm aware of nothing else. I realized many years ago that I had better not arrange to do anything else during an interview, like turn off an appliance or make a telephone call, as I would always forget. At other times my memory for such tasks was fine, but during a session with a client, I have turned my mind to engaging him and his problem totally. Diagnosis and treatment is guesswork without having engaged the client's subconscious, otherwise the therapist is still dealing with the client's defended intellectual appreciation of his gout or his Crohn's disease. By treating such a version of his illness, both practitioner and client remain in the same defended frame of reference, that is, the condition is beyond the control of the individual. Symptom relief is often the only acceptable treatment to the conscious mind. The trance state allows the therapist to diagnose the needs and advantages behind the client's decision to have the illness. The doctor allows his own subconscious to diagnose for him. This frees him from having to sift through a great deal of irrelevant material that both he and the client will raise in order to feel safe. The client's investment in remaining superficial about his disease is his fear of change, while the doctor will be tempted to keep the client sick in order to feel needed.

The trance state is not the deep trance that many of us associate with the antics of stage hypnotists, it is simply that state of concentration that excludes all else beyond the immediate task at hand. We have all experienced it, perhaps the most obvious example being when we are watching a movie or reading a book. When something else takes our attention we "snap out of it," and are often surprised at how occupied we've been. Often a long time has passed of which we are totally unaware. "Gracious, is that the time!" we say to ourselves, having sat up for hours longer than we intended watching a thriller on TV. Other times that we experience the trance state are at the moment of falling asleep and waking each day, or at work when our mind "wanders," the well-known state of reverie. These are all hypnotic states, self-induced, and are similar to the frame of mind in which my client and I engage each other. If either of us is afraid of the other, the state of trance will not be achieved, and we will both know that the majority of the problem remains. In a few more sessions we may resolve it.

PICKING A GOOD DOCTOR

This is easy, since there's no such thing as a good or a bad doctor, just doctors who are right for you at a particular time. When, or if, your original choice no longer suits you, you can change your original contract with the doctor, or change doctors. If you allow yourself to follow your feelings and intuition, you will automatically pick someone who has a similar appreciation of your disease. If you're too frightened to pick a doctor by such a method, you stay where you are until it's safer for you to move. Then you risk a little.

If the doctor believes that tonsillitis is caused by a streptococcus, and that penicillin will cure it, and you also choose to believe that, you'll be attracted to each other. After your child has suffered three attacks of tonsillitis during the one winter, and had three courses of antibiotics, and your doctor still maintains that upper respiratory tract inflammations are caused by organisms and that the solution is to take more antibiotics, you may decide to seek a second opinion. Most likely you'll be offered the opportunity to discuss the matter with an ear, nose and throat surgeon, with the same explanation, but a different treatment, namely removing the tonsils or, if the middle ear is a complication, inserting tubes through the tympanic membranes. If you call "Halt, I no longer trust your appreciation of my child's disease, I'm going to seek an alternative approach," you may find a clinical dietitian who removes all dairy products from the child's diet and supplements it with calcium-containing vegetables. In addition the dietitian may add more raw green vegetables, increase the fiber in the diet to regulate the bowels and remove some of the simple, rapidly absorbed sugars. If you trust this woman, and believe her treatment makes sense, you'll pass that belief through your words and actions to your child who, if he similarly chooses to believe, will recover and stop having tonsillitis or middle ear infections.

Or you may decide that since the child develops the ear infections only when his father returns to his job on the oil rig, where he's away for two months at a time, the basis of the problem is psychological. The child is giving himself ear infections in order to keep his father at home, or perhaps to attract greater support from his mother while he is absent. In this case you may take the family to see a family therapist, who reassures the child that even though his father is away from home he still loves the child, and that his mother will care for him while he's gone. Dad may choose to telephone home or write to the boy more often. When the child no longer needs the ear infections he'll stop them.

Medical practice is a supply and demand industry. If more people require dietetic advice, then more dietitians will become available. Naturopaths, if more people require naturopathic treatment, will proliferate. Similarly, osteopathy, chiropractic, radionics, radiaesthesia, herbalism, Gestalt, Primal Scream, Transactional Analysis, radix, neo-Reichian bodywork, drug therapy, surgery, bio-energetics, hypnotherapy, acupuncture, Rolfing, homeopathy, color therapy, massage, psychoanalysis, transpersonal psychology, JEL, est, Ayurvedic, visualization, flower remedies, behavior modification and encounter will all be patronized by people to whom they appeal at the time. It's wonderful to have a choice.

LEARNING FROM ILLNESS

When I attend a practitioner, one of my main concerns is to find out to what extent her particular discipline is capable of teaching me how to care for myself. Will I need to attend this practitioner regularly for the rest of my life, with no insight into my illness, or will I learn from her how to keep myself well in the future? If she offers no insight as to how I prevent my current illness recurring, or how I prevent other illness from developing, then I'm not interested. In my quest to be responsible for myself, I don't want to remain dependent upon the expertise of a practitioner who cannot or will not explain what is happening, and who won't teach me how to take care of myself. Illness is to be learned from, and if the discipline you first choose to treat a problem fails to enlighten you, and you wish to know why you have made yourself ill and how to increase your options for becoming well, I advise you to seek an alternative. People who are on a course of self-discovery and self-responsibility will find little joy in contemporary orthodox medical practice. You can't learn much in the ten minutes it takes to have a drug prescribed. The drug simply suppresses the physical and psychological symptoms, thereby decreasing rather than increasing awareness of the problem. Those not wishing to care for themselves will, however, find excellent symptomatic relief, and, if they're keen to lose any organs, willing accomplices. If they hurt themselves in a vehicular accident, they'll be helped by one of modern medicine's greatest technical achievements, reconstructive surgery.

Illness provides an opportunity for us to grow. I have proposed the notion that we give ourselves illnesses in order to take care of more frightening psychological needs. If we discard the usual medical model that there's something "wrong" with us, and it should be abated with a drug, or cut out with a knife, and instead regard illness as an integral part of the growth process, we will have a clearer notion of its value. By the indiscriminate removal of a disease process, we have not removed something that was making us unhappy, we have removed something that was taking care of us. When we realize this, we can begin to use illness effectively. One can no more abandon an illness than one can abandon a part of our experience. We can no more cure illness by denying it than we can deny that we were once five years old. We cure ourselves by accepting it and by then choosing another option, different from the illness we originally chose. The disease then becomes part of our experience, able to draw upon at any time. We can revive it if necessary, or leave it dormant. Imagine going to a surgeon and saying, "I want you to cut out my experience between the ages of two and four, since it was a particularly traumatic time for me, and I want to forget it." Disease and learning are part of life.

As you read this book I wonder if you related any of what has been said to your own situation. Perhaps you've been adopting the position of a detached observer, learning how other people "give themselves illness" while you "catch" yours. Or perhaps you've felt guilty at having given yourself a disease, and consider yourself weak to have been afraid to ask for the caring that you wanted directly, rather than suffering. I repeat, everything you've so far done you've done to care for yourself, and is sensible, honorable and, if need be, remediable. If you want to examine any illness from which you're currently suffering, or from which you've suffered in the past, using the frame of reference with which you're now familiar, ask yourself the following questions.

HOW HAS YOUR ILLNESS CHANGED:

1. The way you are feeling? (What were you feeling before becoming ill, and what are you feeling now?)
2. The way you are thinking? (What were you thinking before becoming ill, and what are you thinking now?)
3. The way you are feeling about yourself?
4. The way you are feeling about life generally?
5. Your feelings towards others?

6. The relationship between you and your spouse, lover, partner, children, father, mother, siblings, other family?
7. Your ability to work?
8. The way you feel about work?
9. Your relationship with your workmates?
10. Your relationship with your boss?
11. Your employment prospects?
12. Your mobility?
13. Your financial state?
14. Your ability to play sport?
15. Your ability to travel?
16. Your self-worth?
17. Your ability to have sex with your partner?
18. Your ability to have sex with others?
19. Your ability to care for yourself, your spouse, your children, others?
20. Your need to be looked after?
21. Your ability to be independent?
22. Your ability to be happy?
23. Your willingness to be adventurous?
24. Your willingness to make it?
25. Your will to live?

Now that you are aware of how your illness is responsible for changing the way you feel, think and act, turn the whole notion of cause and effect upside down. "How has your illness caused the way you feel, think and act?" becomes "How has the way you feel, think and act caused your illness?"

The way you feel, think and act, and your illness, are both a consequence of your personality. They are both the result of early childhood decisions—one does not "cause" the other. The notion that because we are ill, certain things take place, serves the purpose of:

1. Removing responsiblity from us ("If it weren't
   for this cold, I would . . . ")
2. Confirming our fears ("Damn gonorrhea, it'll be
   a long time before I have sex again . . . ")
3. Justifying our feelings, thoughts and actions to
   ourselves and to others ("I'd really love to go to
   Bavaria next Christmas, but the cold climate
   doen't suit my bronchitis . . . ")

If we consider the end result of our being ill, we'll
discover what we've set out (often in our subconscious)
to achieve. We have changed our lives, using the illness to do it. We create the illness and in turn invest
in it the power to change our lives. Illness, alone, is
impotent. For example, a cold is not some unlucky
event that prevents us from working. We give ourselves a cold in order to stop work. Arthritis is not
some unfortunate disease which destroys our independence. We are scared to be independent so we give
ourselves arthritis. Cancer is not something we develop by chance. It's something we give ourselves
when we're too scared to live. People don't die. They
kill themselves. Sometimes having illness *is* the best
way of getting what we want. Health involves a willingness to take responsiblity for the decision to be ill.

The following exercise in guided imagery will clarify some of the advantages in you being ill. Either
read it yourself, or have someone read it to you, paus-
ing where appropriate.

Quiet your mind, release those things you've been
concentrating on in this room, make yourself comfortable in your chair, take three or four deep breaths,
blow out the tensions from your body, and relax. Cast
your mind back to the last time that you were ill, to
the place where you were ill, to the house or hospital

and to the room you were lying in, and be there for a moment in that place, lying quietly. And see that place and the things about you as you lie there, hear the sounds, smell the smells, notice the movements of the trees outside the window or the cars in the street.

See yourself lying there or sitting in your chair and become aware of this ill person who is you. As you lie there, let yourself be aware of how you're feeling, if you have pain, or discomfort, whether you're quiet or restless, hot or cold, breathing easily or with difficulty, or any other bodily sensations you may have. And as you lie there, let yourself become aware of your feelings, whether or not you're sad, or afraid, or angry, bitter or resentful, whether you're joyful, excited or anything else you're feeling as you are ill.

Now become aware, if you haven't already done so, of the other people who are there with you, while you're ill, either with you continually or intermittently. See their faces, see what's there, and hear what they're saying to you or to others who may be in the room. And as you become aware of their presence, be aware of anyone else who you would like to be there who is not. If there's someone who you would especially like to be with you while you're ill, put them there. Allow yourself to experience what they're doing and saying, and how you're feeling about them and others who are either present or absent. And as you experience being ill and the people in your life who are important to you at this time, be aware of what you're telling yourself about this illness, or others you've had, and how you're reacting to being unwell. Become aware of what you think about being ill, how you regard yourself as a person now that you're ill and what you know about people who are ill.

Leaving your illness for the moment, find yourself

on a beautiful day with the sun shining, walking across a green meadow with the air fresh and the sky blue. At the end of the meadow is a path leading towards a small house, and as you walk through the meadow along the path towards the house, you can see something written on the door of the house. As you get closer you can see the words "ADVANTAGES FROM BEING ILL." Now open the door and let come out just one of the advantages in being ill that are within the house, knowing that the ones which are just inside the door, and which come out first, are the safest for you to consider first. Now talk to the advantage that you've let out and get to know it, letting the advantage tell you how this illness that you have has really been helping you in some way. And as you talk with it, find out about the good things you've been getting, which may be anything at all, for the house has thousands of varied advantages.

Now thank your illness for looking after you so well. And as you thank your illness, you may like to ask how else you could have come to get the good things for yourself without needing to go through the uncomfortable things like the aches and pains and miseries of the illness. Be aware that at this point in time you may be willing to get what you want in other ways, or you may choose to not remove the illness at this time, and do so later. The decision is yours.

Allow yourself to experience some of the things you're not getting in your life at the moment that you would like, and see if they are related in any way to your illness, or if your advantage in having the illness gets those things for you. Consider this awhile. And now say goodbye to the advantage that you took out of the house and know that it, and the illness, will be there, within the house, if you want them. And as you walk back down the path through the meadow with the sun shining warmly down upon you, and the breeze blowing warmly and gently, let yourself feel the new power of the things you've discovered. Be with yourself for a few moments longer, feeling what you will, and then come back here to this room, to the book you are reading, and relax a moment with yourself.

When you're ready, you may like to turn back a few pages and reconsider the questions on page 364. "How has your illness changed?":

1.
2.
3.

ILLNESS AND SOCIETY

I've stated previously that illness is partly an anthropological matter. Societies need illnesses in similar ways to individuals, that is, they are the result of social scripting as well as personal scripting. The role that illness plays will vary between and within societies, as in individuals, with their needs. Historical, geographical, genetic and social factors all determine that diseases of one society will differ from diseases elsewhere. The significance of the various factors will vary. Poor hygiene, nutrition and a dusty environment will be more important in the development of trachoma in the Australian Aboriginal than a racial need for an eye complaint. Similarly, working in coal mines may be more causative of anthracosis, and working in asbestos plants more causative of asbestosis, than a need on the part of the workers for a lung condition. And yet many people are exposed to these environmental pollutants and don't develop disease. We have discussed previously how these individuals protect themselves against disease by having no need for illness. Collectively, as in the case of the miners, they may force management to improve the working environment. Societies may also live under similar conditions, but have different illness profiles. It's well documented in medical literature that the incidence of diseases differs across societies, and although environmental and dietetic explanations exist for these differences, I believe that the condoning of various diseases and the rejecting of others is an equally powerful factor.

Would you rather tell someone that you were suffering from arthritis or veneral disease? Would you rather tell someone you had a cold sore on the lip or genital herpes? They are virtually the same organism. What illness do you have that you're quite willing to tell others about; and do you have others that you're less willing to discuss? Your answer is likely to reflect the image you have of yourself, and also the social pressures that condone certain diseases and not others.

If you kill yourself, then a vehicle accident or cancer is more socially acceptable than suicide. If you want people to respect your suffering, then arthritis is more effective than irritable-bowel syndrome, being more visible. Society condones minor upper-respiratory infections (they are a national pastime), and rejects people who choose to go mad instead, even though they may have the same needs (time out with caring). As governments and their social services take more responsibility for us (the carrot we are offered in order to accede to their wishes), diseases are increasingly being used to facilitate the hand-over of power to an outside person or agency. Often we're willing to be relieved of the burden of self-responsiblity as quickly as possible. The government instrumentalities in turn foster an atmosphere of non-individual responsiblity, and actively encourage people to become unwell and dependent. By so doing they increase their stranglehold on people's lives. Imagine what would happen if people decided that they were not going to become seriously ill. The medical hierarchy, the drug companies, the insurance companies and a large part of the public service would all be out of work. These bodies are among the most influential in our society. Your health is not necessarily in their best interests.

Illness is commonly deployed to avoid unwanted emotions. The less willing a society is to outwardly express anger, sadness, joy and fear, the more common this particular usage of disease will be. Take the following situation.

The foreman on a busy production line is genuinely concerned about the dangerous working environment. Driven by his own scripting to be responsible for others, he works at improving conditions on the factory floor. Management treats him warily, realizing both his potential to increase production and to stop it altogether. The workers use him to improve both their pay and conditions. Despite considerable headway in that which he set out to achieve, he finds he's no happier than before. The workers never seem satisfied and management distrusts him, blaming him for poor productivity and industrial unrest. He becomes very frustrated, has increasing doubts about his self-worth, becomes chronically afraid, develops kidney failure and is forced to retire. Both management and workers make speeches about his great work, and both pay spe-

cial attention to his efforts in the field of industrial re-
lations. He receives a golden handshake and, much to
the relief of everyone, invalids himself out of their
lives. He changes residence so that he may be further
from them and nearer the dialysis machine at the
hospital.

Illness has facilitated the resolution of a difficult
social situation. In other societies, the workers and
the management may have had a more respectful relationship; as a child the foreman may not have been
raised to care for others; the retirement through illness may not have attracted a financial reward; the
wife may have not been interested in caring for a sick
partner; the hospital may or may not have had money
donated by a drug company with which to buy a dialysis machine; and the foreman may have been prepared
to withstand the attempts of both parties to use him.
In that case this scenario wouldn't have developed. All
of the factors influencing the expression and timing of
this man's illness were, to a degree, socially determined. To that same degree the illness itself was socially determined.

In the capitalistic world, money is often behind one
group of people encouraging others to become ill. The
drug companies are uniquely poised to exert pressure
on governments to spend money in one area or another. They are, however, no more responsible for what
has happened than anyone else. It's nonsense to blame
them. They've responded to the market place, to the
call by the people for more and more powerful
symptom-relieving drugs. In this they've been aided
by a medical profession ready and willing to promote
any system of medicine, which effectively maintains
the status quo, that is, the patient loses his symptoms,

keeps his disease, learns nothing and pays dearly for all three. The doctor remains overworked, defensive, powerful and, if he wants, wealthy.

Economically, it's very much better in the long run to have people take responsiblity for themselves, and to stop regarding illness as bad luck and therefore warranting financial reimbursement. Illness is such an integral part of our society, and such a pillar of our financial system, that I don't hold much hope of changing it. Nor do I necessarily want to. I raise it here as an option. Take, for example, the average course of events in any number of general practices all over the country.

Thousands of general practitioners see hundreds of thousands of patients superficially every day. They may send a fifth of these people to specialists, often not because the general practitioner lacks skills, but because they don't have the time to diagnose and treat them properly. If a doctor sees many patients in a day, he can earn about four times as much money as he can if he sees fewer people but deals with them in depth. Very few doctors choose the latter option. Those patients sent off to specialists, for which the insurance funds, that is, you and I, pay, are likely to be further investigated, since that's part of specialist medical practice. EKGs, blood tests, X-rays, scans, endoscopy, surgical procedures and so on are all generated by the specialist practitioner. Then hospitals, para-medical care, recovery and rehabilitation all play a part, not to mention the drugs that are almost invariably prescribed. The income generated by the one client attending the general practitioner, and being superficially dealt with, is enormous. If the general practitioner, or the practitioner of first contact, were remunerated for doing the job properly in the first place, there would be minimal expense. In addition, the client could be taught how to avoid future illness in himself and his family and even greater savings made.

To effect such changes in medical practice would mean an enormous change in perspective on the part of the public, the government and the medical fraternity, including alternative practitioners. As it stands, governments are pressured into buying the latest technological advances that keep the powerful hospital specialists happy, and are of little or no benefit to the majority of people paying for them. The cost of new medical technology is phenomenal. With each new multi-million dollar "advance" comes a decrease in the reliance that the public puts on common sense and its own ability to heal itself. The fear generated by the implication that "anyone who doesn't have a yearly scan is running the risk of cancer" causes far more deaths than it saves lives. Multiphasic screening is making some people very rich and guaranteeing the illness of the gullible. We can believe that the machines, laboratory tests, drugs and medical insurance will keep us well, or believe instead that we can make and keep ourselves well. The former belief will eventually bankrupt us all. The latter will result in cost-effective technical and psychological support for people intent on healing themselves.

As society evolves, so does its appreciation of those things which ail it. It's a mistake to believe that because we understand anatomy, physiology and biochemistry better than we ever have, we understand more about human beings and our diseases. Rather do we understand them differently. Our explanation of the things that happen to our minds and bodies will depend on the metaphor of the day. The metaphor of the day depends on the general direction of society. Let me give an example.

Since the Industrial Revolution, our metaphor has become increasingly mechanical. The heart isn't *pumping* properly. The liver, which is like a complex *chemical factory*, is malfunctioning. The *acid erosion* of the protective layer of the stomach results in a stomach ulcer. With increasing technological sophistication, particularly since the Second World War, the tendency to attribute malfunctions of the body to mechanical breakdown has increased. This means that the origins of disease, and the treatment of disease, will also be regarded as mechanical. We now think of illness in technological, mechanical terms. The mechanical concept of disease isn't the only concept of disease, nor the correct concept. Neither is it incorrect. It's simply one notion of disease, based on the current metaphor. It happens to be the concept of disease which suits, or has suited, the industrial society.

Knowing the basis of our notions of disease, it isn't difficult to see how our two major therapies, chemical therapy (drugs) and mechanical therapy (surgery), have arisen. It's also easy to see why other concepts of illness are rejected, using fear and ignorance masquerading as logic. The logic holds only within the narrow, mechanical frame of reference.

People hoped, as they always have, that the current metaphor, and the notions stemming from it, would make them happy. Technological medicine was to have healed the world of all disease by now. Instead we have simply replaced the old diseases with new ones, or revived those that we temporarily shelved. The belief that drugs will save us is passing. Our belief that the technologists will heal us is lying in tatters on the surgery floor.

The Industrial Revolution is being replaced by the Personal Revolution. The notion of disease as the mechanical failing of a machine under duress is being replaced by the notion that disease is the physical manifestation of internal conflicts. The change from one idea to the other isn't new. It's happened no doubt many times before and will happen again. Those in the forefront of medicine are not those who will devise something new but those who see change as inevitable, imminent and see it early. Disease will be regarded as a personal decision. This change is made more necessary by the financial strictures of the technological revolution. It's simply impossible to continue funding the old-style medicine. People have to take more responsibility and therefore more care of themselves. When society has made the next great leap forward, my concept of disease, depending as it does on emerging metaphor and my own internal processes, will be archaic. Then it will be the broken idols of psychotherapy that lie gathering dust on the group room floor.

Epilogue

At the start of the wet season above the plains a long way from the coast, a tiny rivulet is given life. Gathering every available tributary, it struggles in those harsh regions for survival. The trees, unable to sustain themselves from such a small creek, have not troubled to establish themselves along its barely green edges. Nor do fish or animals rely on the meager water supply for their own needs, knowing its inconstancy. The sun makes moderate demands, evaporating a small portion of that water, which has not sought refuge by running underground.

The terrain is a dominant influence in the infancy of the creek. The fledgling waters, in order to keep gathering, must satisfy the dictates of the land. In the early stages of its life, every rise, no matter how small, must be negotiated. Every dip, no matter how shallow, must be filled, before the waters, fed slowly by those following, can begin to move towards the ocean. In such a climate is the small waterway nurtured, fed by the land and, in order to guarantee its survival, aware of all the land exacts.

Epilogue

As the creek becomes surer with time and distance, accumulating the experience of its many tributaries, it begins to acquire its own strength. Larger water-courses join its course, and before long it begins, tentatively at first, to support life about it. Small trees adorn its banks, tadpoles breed in its quiet reaches, and the sun, attesting its permanence, places heavier demands upon its waters. The landscape, once complete master over the course it must flow, is now bargained with. Sometimes the creek defers to the strength of a mountain range, turning back the way it came in order to find an opening, but as it gains in maturity and becomes a river, it makes its own mark upon the countryside.

Forging its way along valley floors and through gorges and canyons, the river changes the face of the land which spawned it. No longer needing to acquiesce for survival to every whim of the terrain, and aware of their mutual need, the river rejoices in its independence by supporting large trees, fish, birds and animals, and supplying small creeks and rock pools with clear water. The sun's ever-increasing demand for evaporation is met with ease.

When the last of the ranges has been negotiated, the river celebrates its course towards the sea, free of the need to rely upon others for its survival. Some of the early meanderings made in order to continue gathering water and appease the terrain are replaced by a graceful and powerful flow towards the ocean. Thankful for having followed the early directions of the land, the river blends with the ocean, feeling the power of achievement, the warmth of co-existence and the exhilaration of freedom. Born of the ocean and traveling the long journey back to the place where they first began, the waters know themselves for the time.

He who understands paradox understands illness. When I say that an individual needs or wants an illness, and insures that he suffers from it, I'm speaking of the paradox inherent within the words need and want. If you ask the person with cancer why he needs cancer, he will tell you that he doesn't need it, want it or like it. And of course, to his knowledge, he's being completely truthful. Nobody likes the aches, pains and anguish of being unwell. If the same person with cancer is offered the option of surviving by confronting his greatest fears, in many cases he will choose the cancer. He needs the cancer to avoid the fear. His decision either way is entirely honorable.

Fear is the basis of all illness. Fear necessitates the early childhood adaptations which result in illness. We are afraid to take responsibility for ourselves. We don't trust our own parent to look after our own child, the grown-up part of us to look after the little kid in us. We try and get someone else to do it for us, for we were never taught in childhood that we could do it ourselves and do it successfully. Our illness confirms our frailty and our need for a caretaker. If, in addition, we don't like our little kid much, then even if we have the skills we may be disinclined to care for him or her. With either attitude we are likely to attract people to us who agree with our dismissal of our own parenting abilities, or don't like the little kid in us much either. Continuing confirmation of our own inadequacy requires continuing incapacity, usually chronic illness.

To cure ourselves we need to take back the responsiblity of loving and caring for our little kids from whomever we have entrusted the task. We need to accept ourselves whoever, whenever and however we are. That means accepting that we have made ourselves unwell in order to care for ourselves the very best we know how. When we have taken back full responsibil-

ity for our little kids, we can find another grown-up
who will be willing to help us look after him or her.
Our little kids can play with each other, while the
grown-ups share the joys and burdens of responsibility.

We can make use of those healing professionals, orthodox or alternative, who make themselves available.
We can pass through the transition stage of partial
responsiblity while under the umbrella of their care.
When we are ready we can risk leaving the nest and
taking off on our own, knowing that we can return if
we want. It is not for me, with my own needs, to tell
you how, when or where you do it. I have suggested a
program for recovery, a program for growth and discovery. Ultimately, your universe is beyond me.

Use this as you will. From here on there is room for
one person only. From a distance I see you standing at
the gate of your soul, looking in. You like very much
what you see.

Bibliography

Berne, E., *Games People Play*, Penguin, New York, 1964.

Berne, E., *What Do You Say After You Say Hello?*, Grove Press, New York, 1972.

British Medical Journal, 1982, 23, p. 284.

Darby, D.N., S. Glasser, and I.F. Wilkinson, *Health Care and Lifestyle*, New South Wales University Press, Sydney, 1981.

Goulding, R., *Changing Lives Through Redecision*, Bruner Mazel, New York, 1979.

Goulding, R., *The Power is in the Patient*, T.A. Press, San Francisco, 1976.

James, M., and D. Jongeward, *Born to Win*, Addison-Wesley, New York, 1971.

Karpman, S., "Fairytale and Script Drama Analysis," *Transactional Analysis Bulletin*, 7, no. 26 (April 1968), pp. 39-43.

Kitzinger, S., *The Experience of Childbirth*, Penguin, Harmondsworth, UK, 1978.

Lankton, S.R., *Practical Magic*, Meta Publications, California, 1980.

Bibliography

Leboyer, F., *Birth Without Violence*, Wildwood House, London, 1975.

Mann, F., *Acupuncture*, Vintage, New York, 1973.

Perls, F., *Gestalt Therapy Verbatim*, Real People Press, Utah, 1969.

Rosenbloom, A., *The Natural Birth Control Book*, Aquarian Research Foundation, Philadelphia, 1977.

Shears, C., *Nutritional Science and Health Education*, Downfield Press, Stroud, UK, 1976.

Simonton, O.C., S. Simonton, and J. Creighton, *Getting Well Again*, Bantam Books, New York, 1980.

Spitz, R., "Hospitalism Genesis of Psychiatric Conditions in Early Childhood," *Psycho-analytic Study of the Child*, vol. 1, 1945, pp. 53-74.

Steiner, C., *Scripts People Live*, Bantam Books, New York, 1974.

Woolams, S., and M. Brown, *Transactional Analysis*, Prentice-Hall, New York, 1979.

Index

If you would like to receive a catalog of products and information about future workshops, lectures and events sponsored by the Louise L. Hay Educational Institute which assists people in loving themselves, please detach and mail the postcard below.

I would like to be placed on the Hay House, Inc. mailing list.

NAME_____

ADDRESS_____

_____

Book in which this card was attached:

_____

HAY HOUSE, INC.
P. O. Box 2212
Santa Monica, CA 90406